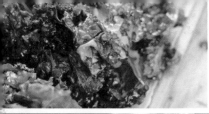
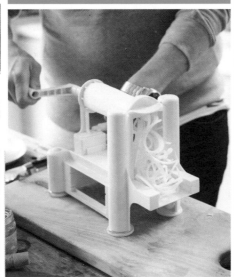
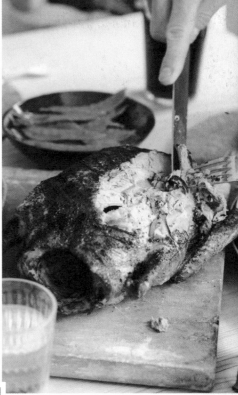
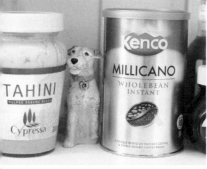
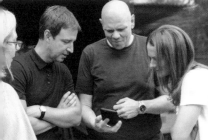
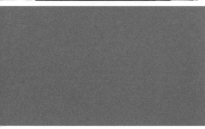
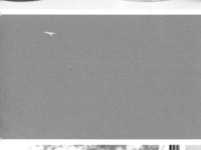
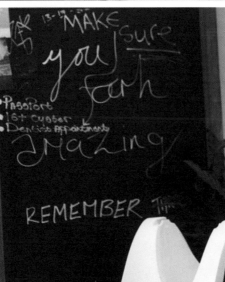
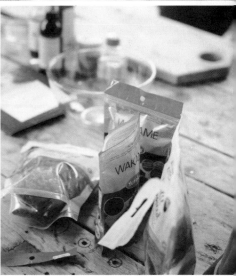
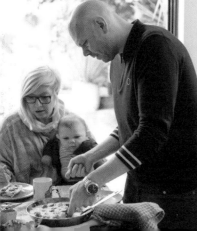
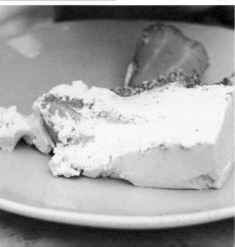

TAHINI

PULPED SESAME SEEDS

Cypressa

Kenco
MILLICANO
WHOLEBEAN
INSTANT

A UNIQUE BLEND OF INSTANT COFFEE
& FINELY-MILLED COFFEE BEANS

MAKE sure
you
earn
- Passport
- 16+ cuoter
- Dentist Appointment
amazing

REMEMBER This

P9-CJJ-754

TOM KERRIDGE'S
DOPAMINE DIET

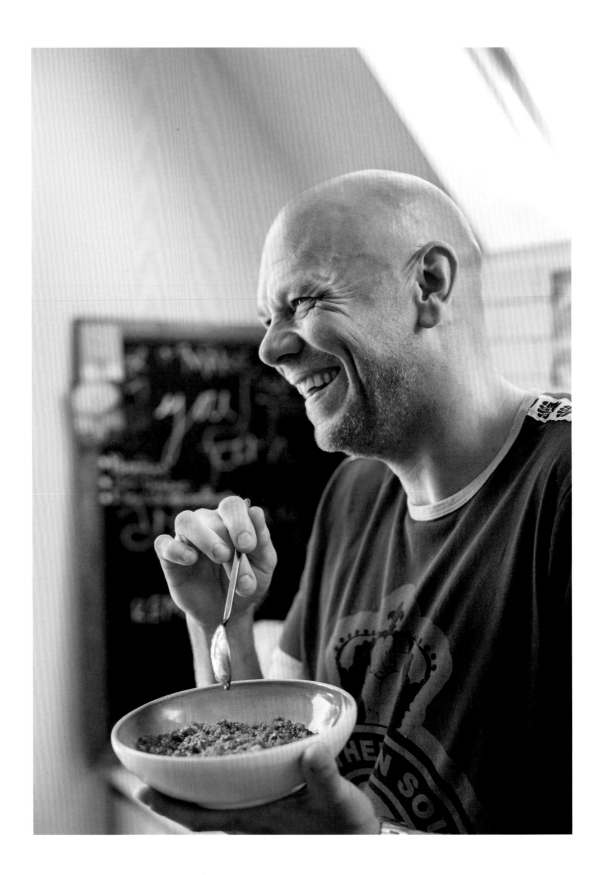

TOM KERRIDGE'S DOPAMINE DIET

My low-carb, stay-happy way to lose weight

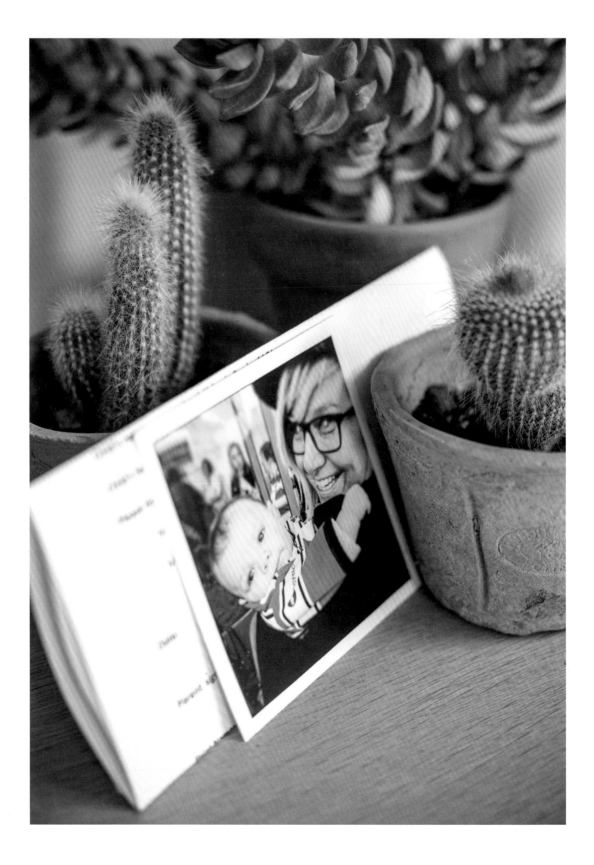

I dedicate this book to Ninja Mum – Bef, you're the best, love you always. And to Acey, the funniest, most amazing and incredible thing to have ever happened in my life, who as I write this is chewing on one of his dirty socks!

CONT

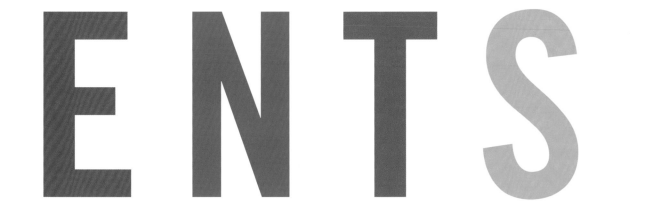

MY DOPAMINE DIET

OVER THE PAST THREE YEARS I've lost eleven stone. As a chef and someone who's constantly on the go, I've always known that I'd only be able to stick to a diet that allows me to eat really delicious food. I started by cutting out booze and then began to devise my own low-carb regime built around ingredients that are known to facilitate the release of dopamine, the 'pleasure hormone'. Thankfully, these include some of my favourite things, such as free-range eggs, good-quality meat, oily fish, artichokes and leafy greens, so I haven't felt deprived or hungry for a minute. Since I've lost so much weight, people always ask me how I did it. The answer is in these pages.

My looming fortieth birthday was a turning point. Even without weighing myself, at a rough guess, I reckon I was nearly 30 stone. When you live a full and busy life, it's easy to ignore the obvious as you frantically try to cram as much as you can into each day. But there's nothing like a major milestone to focus the mind.

I work in an industry full of hard-drinking party animals, and I had built the reputation of being the last man standing at every awards do, party and get-together. My love of booze and late-night food was legendary. But as my birthday approached, I started to think I needed to change. I couldn't continue to live like this.

But in a business that is all about delicious, rich food and limitless drink, how could I begin to make a change and find a weight-reducing regime that was right for me?

Of course, everyone tells you how important exercise is. And I get that, but unless you've walked in my size 10 shoes, it's difficult to imagine just how intimidating it is to go into a gym as a 40-year-old, 30-stone bloke and hand yourself and your health over to some 25-year-old personal trainer with a six pack. Emotionally, physically, you're so far apart there is no common ground. You feel awkward, embarrassed and – particularly challenging for someone like me, who's used to being in charge of everything around them – out of

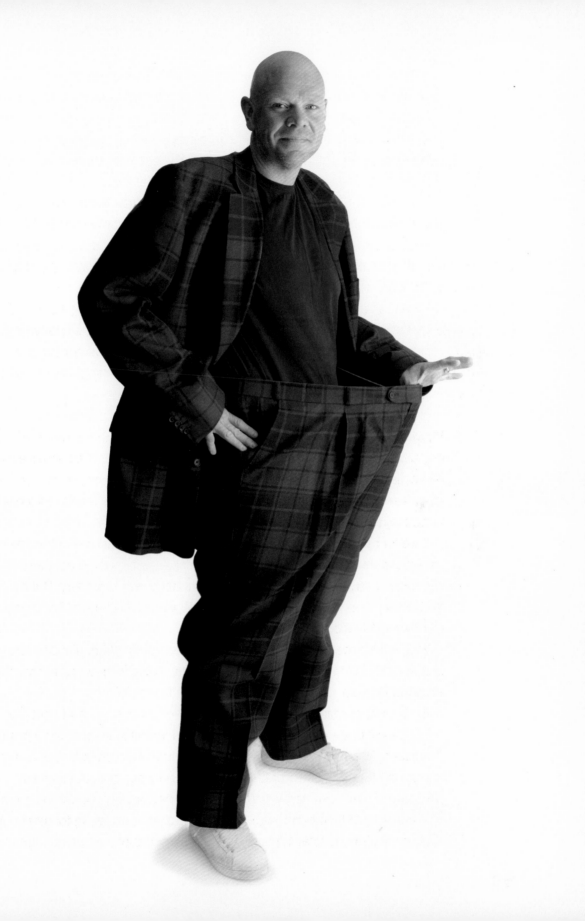

control. I realised that I would have to start with food and gently find my own way into exercise (see page 19). You will find your own way too.

Open any paper or magazine, turn on the telly, or click on the internet, and you are bombarded with diet advice. It's overwhelming and often contradictory. Professors, doctors, nutritionists and all sorts of other experts will tell you that it's about a 'balanced' diet and lifestyle.

I knew that for me – and for anyone who has lots of weight to lose – this wouldn't work. I wasn't going to drop the daunting amount I needed to lose by having one scoop of ice cream instead of two. 'Balance' keeps you the same. 'Balance' is for when you've achieved a weight you're happy with and want to maintain it.

It was clear that to lose a lot of weight my diet had to be *unbalanced*. I am aware this flies in the face of popular diet wisdom, but I knew that at 30 stone, I had to take a really hard look at my life and make a big shift. To reduce my size I would have to remove some of the things that were making me – and keeping me – fat. I needed to think about what my priorities were, what was wrong in my diet, and what I needed to take away to get the results I wanted.

I spent ages researching diets and trying to find inspiration for something that would work for me. I read everything I could get my hands on. I looked at calorie counting, fat-free diets and protein-led regimes. I even considered quirky ingredient diets like the 'cabbage soup diet'. At one point, I thought I'd find out if there was such a thing as a beer diet, so I could eradicate food and just drink beer. (Sadly, that doesn't exist.)

None of the existing regimes seemed right for me – they were too fussy, too restrictive or just plain unpleasant. So it was back to the drawing board. I knew my situation could not be solved with a quick-fix, two-month fad diet. It was important for me to find something I could stick to in the long term, a style of eating I wouldn't get bored with after a few weeks before sliding back into my old, bad boy ways. I needed to find something that could become a way of life.

I realised pretty quickly that calorie counting wasn't for me. Even though I could still eat the foods I wanted, I feared I just wouldn't be able to eat enough to satisfy my hunger and fairly quickly I would fall into the habit of having a sneaky something. And then another sneaky something.

Following a fat-free diet would prove very difficult because of my job. Butter, dairy and animal fats are in high use in both of my pubs and, as all chefs and good cooks know, fat carries flavour. How could I sign up for a diet that reduced how good your food could taste? Especially when I was well aware that a bit of butter or a splash of really good olive oil could make all the difference?

So next up, I looked at a low-carbohydrate diet and tried to understand how that works. It quickly became clear to me that a traditional way of eating, even if it's 'balanced', is high in carbohydrates, which increases insulin production, and which in turn leads to more fat accumulation.

I looked at my menu at The Hand and Flowers and saw that one of our best-selling main courses is steak and chips. Hardly surprising – it's lush! Under a low-calorie or low-fat diet, I wouldn't be able to eat this at all. But on a low-carb diet, I realised I could eat at least 50 per cent of it. This is when I knew I was getting somewhere.

As I came to understand the low-carb diet, I realised I could have double steak, no chips, or swap the chips for a side order of vegetables from the menu, such as cabbage, spinach or sprout tops. I could eat out (or in my own restaurant) without feeling like the odd one out. Result!

Also, and significantly, I discovered that swapping bland white carbs for leafy greens has another advantage. Those side dishes are high in iron and have strong, huge, flavours that leave you feeling very satisfied and banish cravings. More about this later…

PUSHING THE PROTEIN, CUTTING OUT CARBS

Once I understood the steak and chips (or rather steak and no chips) theory, I decided to take this approach to everything I ate. I knew that whatever plan I devised, I needed to stay on it long term. I'm easily distracted and I'll happily turn to something new, so I wanted to find a way of eating that would always seem to be the best. It wouldn't work if I became unsatisfied or bored. It had to be as rich, varied and delicious as I could make it.

With this in mind, I knew that a high-protein, high-meat, full-flavoured diet definitely interested me. I knew it could provide enough variety to stop me getting bored, which meant, most importantly, I would be able to stick to it for the long haul. After all, if you can eat pork scratchings on a diet and still lose weight, surely that's a good thing, right?

I don't want to dwell too much on what I don't eat. The reason this has worked so brilliantly for me is because I focus on all of the amazing foods I *can* eat but I realise that, starting out, it's helpful to have a checklist of things to avoid. I cut from my diet all potatoes, pasta, bread, cakes and any of the white, starchy, carb foods that bulk out so much of what we eat.

Carbohydrates are simply a source of energy, which break down into two kinds: starchy foods such as bread and pasta and potatoes, and sugars such as the ones that naturally occur in fruit (fructose) and some dairy (lactose). Some high-fibre foods such as flaxseed contain carbs, but they aren't digested in the same way as highly processed 'white carbs', so they don't negatively impact your blood sugar levels (see page 23).

So spaghetti bolognese became just bolognese (and a delicious one too, see page 150). I still have curry – of course I do! – but no rice, poppadoms or chapatis. If I'm craving something to mop up the sauce, I have my own flatbreads (page 259), containing low-carb coconut flour. Otherwise I have a drier, spicy dish such as piri piri chicken (page 206) or roasted spiced leg of lamb (page 218).

I eat enough to satisfy me, to fill me up, and I don't miss the starchy sides at all. Let's face it, if you were given the choice between ordering rice or tandoori chicken, surely you would opt for the chicken? After all, that's the main event!

I admit, at first it can be a little bit tricky to navigate your way through this, but it's all in the mind. It's natural for us to associate bolognese sauce with pasta, curry with rice, or roast beef with roast potatoes. We've been eating like that for years, so it takes a little while to reprogramme yourself to change your expectations. You're teaching yourself a brand new habit, but once you've got the hang of it, you won't find it difficult.

In fact, the rewards are so immediate and delicious, I promise you it isn't a hardship at all. Immediately, I started really enjoying the food I was eating. I looked for every opportunity to add flavour, to make things taste more intense, and that was enhanced because I had removed the dulling, beige effect of serving everything with pasta, potatoes, bread or rice.

So, full English breakfasts, large omelettes with cheese and bacon, all kinds of chopped salads with spicy chorizo, salty anchovies, feta and olives, have become the staples of my weekday diet. I really cram in flavour and, importantly, texture, wherever I can.

My weekend 'go to' dishes are now meaty, savoury casseroles and stews, which often include umami-rich mushrooms, and slow-roasted joints of meat with crispy skin – whether that be crackling from pork, or the crunchy outside of a shoulder of lamb. I don't miss the crisp, chewy appeal of carby roast

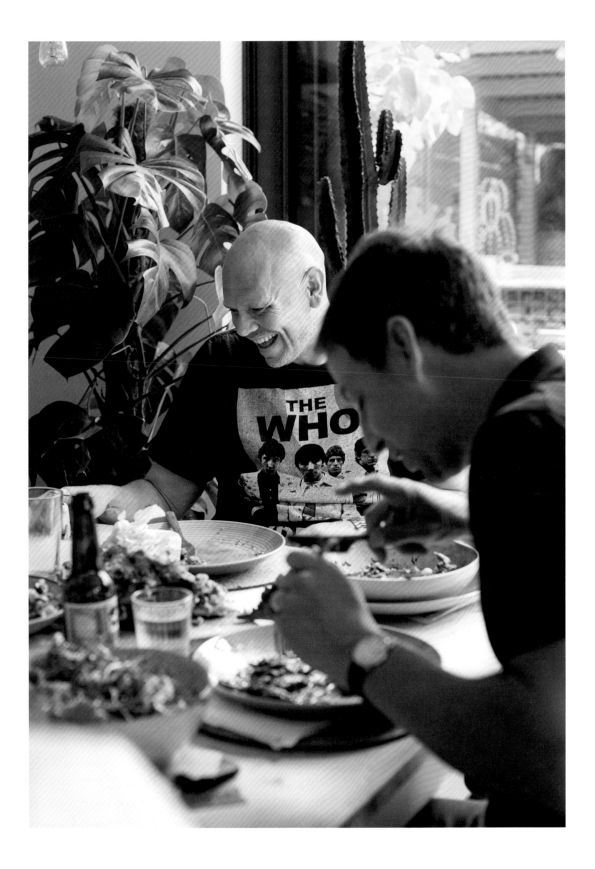

potatoes because I get that lovely mouthfeel in abundance from roasted meats, or even from crisp-skinned fish.

But even I don't eat meat every single day of the week. It's important to balance out your diet with loads of gorgeous vegetables too, and there are plenty of salads and side dishes in this book which will inspire you on those non-meat days.

THE ROLE OF DOPAMINE

When I started to examine my new high-protein/low-carb diet, I wasn't as interested in how it worked nutritionally as I was in why I enjoyed it so much. To me, this is absolutely the key to its success. Everybody else I've ever met moans that diets are a pain and a struggle, but I honestly enjoy mine. I could not have kept going for so long if I didn't. And keeping going is important. I may have lost a lot of weight, but I'd like to lose some more.

This is a long-term project for me – as perhaps it is for you too – and I need lots of variety to keep me motivated. When I reach the weight I want to be, perhaps then I'll consider occasionally returning to some of the foods I've removed from my diet, but I can honestly say that for now, I don't really miss them.

At the very heart of what I have been doing in the past three years is the ethos of eating as many foods which help stimulate the production of dopamine as I can. I'm sure it's this that has kept me up, happy and moving forward with my weight loss.

So what is dopamine? Stay with me. It's a key chemical assisting with neural signalling in the brain's reward hub. To put it simply, when you experience a pleasurable sensation – whether it's from food, laughter, sex, alcohol or gambling – dopamine is released in your brain. There's evidence that suggests low dopamine levels can lead to decreased motivation and make us feel lethargic and apathetic, even depressed – absolutely not the state you need to be in to lose weight.

Dopamine doesn't just appear magically in our brains. Our bodies create it by breaking down an amino acid called tyrosine, which can be obtained from lots of different – and, fortunately, delicious – foods.

I know it may sound like I'm getting all scientific on you, but trust me on this. In this book, I'm just giving you a load of recipes which are fairly low in carbohydrates and high in tyrosine, so they will help boost dopamine levels in the brain. This means that you will enjoy eating them. It is that easy. Many of the recipes are high in protein, which helps you feel fuller for longer, so you shouldn't feel hungry while you're following my dopamine diet.

I am not claiming this is a traditional balanced diet that's low-calorie, low-fat and all of the things we've been told for years will help make us thin (while we get fatter and fatter). It is a selection of favourite recipes that I've enjoyed over the last three years. Alongside taking exercise and cutting out alcohol, they have helped me lose a huge amount of weight without once feeling hungry or deprived. This proof really is in the pudding – but sadly there aren't many of them.

DOPAMINE HEROES

My eating regime has been rich in the following foods over the past couple of years. They are high in the amino acid tyrosine (and its cousin phenylalanine), which can help the body to produce dopamine.

Dairy products I use full-fat cheese, cottage cheese, wholemilk yoghurt and double cream.

Eggs For reasons of welfare and flavour, I always buy organic or free-range eggs. The eggs from chickens raised organically are preferable.

Fish Oily fish, such as salmon, sea bass, trout, tuna, sardines and mackerel, are high in beneficial omega-3 fatty acids and are a good source of vitamin D. Seafood, especially oysters, are also rich in essential omega-3s.

Fruit Apples, bananas, blueberries, grapes, oranges, papaya, strawberries and watermelons are great favourites with me. And yes, I'm aware that these are also quite high in carbohydrates, but they're better than reaching for a burger or a Mars bar if you need a quick fix. Apples, berries and bananas also contain a flavonoid antioxidant called quercetin, which is believed to help the brain prevent dopamine loss.

Well-sourced meat I buy grass-fed beef and lamb, free-range pork and free-range chicken and turkey. It's always worth asking your butcher where his meat comes from.

Nuts Almonds, hazelnuts, pecans and walnuts are among my favourites.

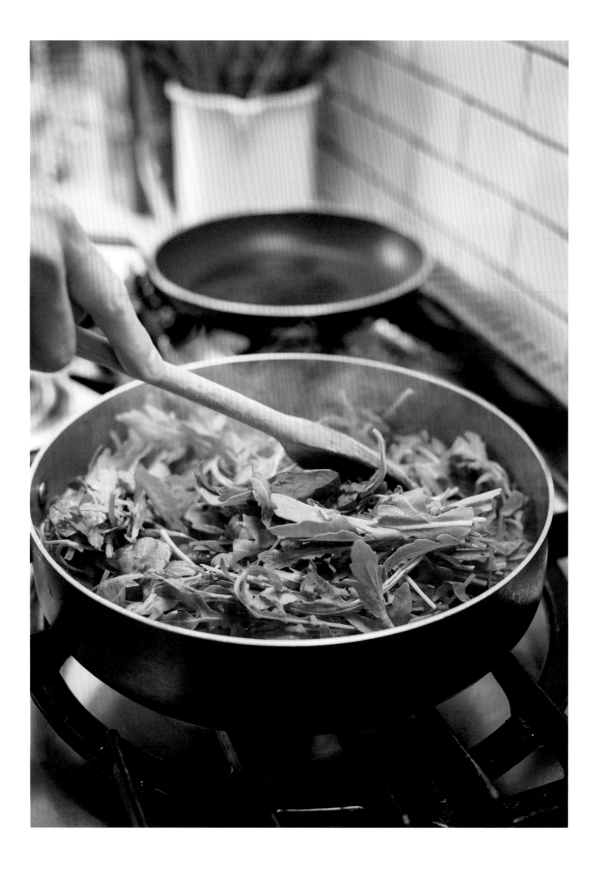

Vegetables My recipes include artichokes, avocados, beetroot, broccoli, cabbage, cauliflower and seaweed such as dulse, wakame, arame and kombu. I particularly love dark green leaves, such as spinach, sprout tops and kale. Their strong, iron-y flavour – especially when combined with grated garlic, salted anchovies and a bit of lemon zest – is incredibly powerful, and as an added bonus, the iron helps to increase dopamine levels. These days, I enjoy greens more than chips, honest!

Spices and chillies I've always loved spicy food, and never more so than now. Hot, chilli-rich foods don't actually increase dopamine levels but they do help to release endorphins in your brain. When you eat hot, spicy food, your mouth sends signals to your brain telling it that it's on fire. Your brain releases endorphins, the body's natural painkiller, which leaves you with a natural 'high'. This is very similar to the feeling that long-distance runners, cyclists and heavy gym users have, when their exertions cross over from pain to pleasure. That's why so many of the recipes in this book have a high chilli and spice content – not just because they're delicious, but because they'll keep you going, keep you up and happy, as you continue to lose weight.

Miscellaneous Chocolate, green tea, vanilla, lavender, sesame seeds and the algae dietary supplement spirulina also help to promote the release of dopamine and endorphins.

Not all dopamine-promoting foods are equal, though! Want to know why we all sometimes crave a cheap burger or can scoff a whole packet of biscuits in a sitting? It's because you get a dopamine buzz from some additives, artificial sweeteners, sugars and junk foods that contain simple carbohydrates, such as burgers, pizzas and cookies. Lots of these foods have an addictive effect on the brain, similar to powerful drugs like cocaine.

Simply put, our brains don't know the difference between a beautiful, dopamine-enhancing chicken, apple and almond salad and a cheap burger that's also dopamine-enhancing. We need to combat the addictive pull of junk food by finding things that raise our dopamine levels but which are also good for us – dishes that give us the same enjoyment as eating a burger and fries, followed by a jam doughnut.

I hope I've done that in this book. All diets require willpower and this one is no different, but if you give my recipes a go, I hope you'll find plenty of delicious, good food you'll want to go back to again and again. I do allow myself the odd Diet Coke sometimes, but apart from that I try to steer away from junk food as much as I can. I prefer to get my dopamine boost from other, more tasty and healthy sources.

THE ALCOHOL QUESTION

Bear with me here, as some of you aren't going to like this! I decided very early on that cutting out all alcohol from my diet was something I had to do. Spirits, wine and beer: they're all gone. This isn't just because alcohol is high in calories; it can have a significant negative impact on all of your good intentions too.

I have one of those personalities with a switch, not a dial. There is no such thing as 'a' glass of wine, or 'a' quick pint. For me, that 'one quick glass' often used to end up as a very late night, finished off with opening up the gin. So for me, alcohol had to go.

I admit this takes willpower. But to make a dramatic change to your life you have to do something dramatically different. The most important factors in success are mindset and determination. I know this from my career as a chef. I realised I had to bring this same focus to my attempt to lose the weight and improve my health.

This is how I worked out a scheme that worked for me. I broke drinking down into four stages. This helped me get over the need for a drink, but still allowed me to go out with my friends for meals, or travel abroad with a load of naughty chefs, without feeling sorry for myself or like I was missing out.

Stage 1 This is the point when you miss booze the most. The moment you walk into the bar, or sit down at the table in the restaurant, that first drink. You miss the nice buzz that comes from having a lovely drink in a nice glass: 1–0 to booze.

Stage 2 In the middle of an evening out, the mood is high, a bit euphoric even. By this point, it doesn't matter if you've been drinking or not, you're actually having a very good time: still 1–0 to booze.

Stage 3 At the end of the evening, the time comes when you realise your friends are a mess, people have started arguing, or are making decisions to do really stupid things. You, meanwhile, are benefiting from the clarity that drinking fizzy water and orange juice all night brings. You can see that booze isn't always the best: 1–1, the equaliser.

Stage 4 The next day, you're up bright and early, clear head, cup of coffee in hand, perhaps even made it to the gym or a swimming pool. With a smile on your face, you know the world is a good place. Your friends, on the other hand… bad times! Booze loses: 1–2, you've taken the lead and won!

I remind myself of these four stages constantly. So long as you remember that the next morning, you're the winner, it's easier to get past the initial hurdle at the beginning of the evening when everyone else is starting to drink. And like so many things, the more you do it, the easier it gets.

THE IMPORTANCE OF EXERCISE

There's no way around it, you need to take some exercise, too. But just like the food, you're more likely to stick to it if you find something you love. I swim every day. For you, it might be swimming, cycling, playing squash or tennis, running, or anything else that involves moving about a bit. Try and find something you don't hate and do it every day if you can!

PICK-ME-UPS

Like lots of you, I am on the go all of the time. With my job and way of life, I'm active, at work and doing things for 16–18 hours a day.

Naturally, I find myself tired at times and in search of a pick-me-up. With my new regime, I have had to make an adjustment as to what that can be. It might be something as simple as a bit of leftover roast meat, some whipped feta (see page 65) with a few crudités, or a super quick omelette (such as the one on page 104). Other times, I reach for something instant to get me through. These are the things that work for me when I need a boost – they might work for you too!

Coffee At the beginning of this journey, I looked at low-carb diets which stressed the importance of eliminating caffeine, but I was mad about caffeine and I still am. Caffeine can deplete dopamine so it isn't to be recommended but I love my coffee! It's a stimulant and helps keep me awake. I've included it in my regime and still lost weight, so if you feel the same way then don't feel you need to step away from the espresso machine.

Chocolate Before I embarked on this regime, I never thought I had a sweet tooth. Once I gave up alcohol though, my body started to crave the sugar it was missing from booze and I found I needed to balance that out in some way. Of course, I was avoiding starchy cakes and desserts, so I started to reach for a bar of chocolate when those cravings struck. I realised quite quickly that this wasn't good. If I had to have some chocolate, I made sure it was the best quality I could find and at least 70 per cent cocoa solids. It's relatively low in carbohydrate but still feels like a treat. Eventually, those cravings subside so I find I reach less and less for a bar of chocolate, but I allow myself the odd square now and again without feeling guilty about it.

Fruit This has become a high-priority food for me. I know that fruits are quite high in sugar, and some low-carb diets severely restrict their consumption, but they feel like a healthy treat. And at the beginning at least, not a day went by without me grabbing a handful of grapes, cold from the fridge. They really began to feel like sweet treats. I've also developed a new-found love of apples, enjoying their crunch and flavour. It's a bonus too that some of the fruits lowest in carbohydrates – berries for example, at only 6g per 100g serving – are rich in antioxidants, as well as being delicious.

Pork scratchings I love these. They're a source of protein so they fill you up, and they have that great crunch you sometimes crave when you're on a diet. You can get them all over the place now, quite posh ones too. As a bar snack or just something to keep in the car for when hunger strikes, pork scratchings have replaced crisps for me.

THE ESSENTIAL ROLE OF SEASONING

As a chef, I've always understood the vital role of seasoning and how getting that just right can elevate an ordinary dish to a really fantastic one. But it has become even more important to me as I have changed the way I eat. How I use salt and other seasonings is vital to making the recipes in this book into dishes I really want to enjoy again and again. The rich umami flavourings from soy, seaweed or even crumbly stock cubes have become central to my home cooking.

I find spices even more exciting now – and I found them pretty exciting before, so this is big! I'm not just after some kind of macho hotter-the-better notion either. I love creating layers of rich, spicy flavour which are really

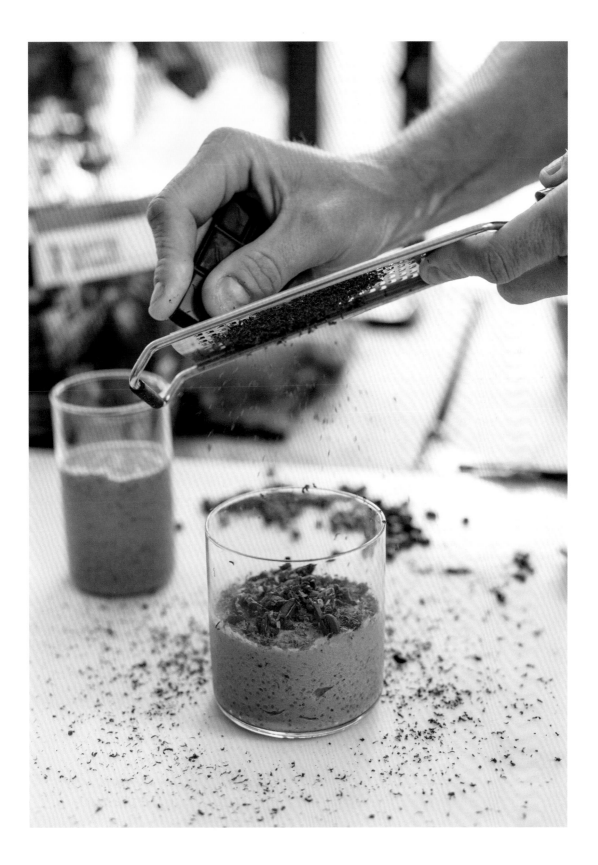

satisfying to eat. Have a go at my slow-roasted shoulder of lamb with mustard glazed greens (page 214) or spiced leg of lamb with cauliflower and coconut (page 218) and you'll see what I mean.

Once I got through the initial three-month period of not just changing the way I eat, but vitally changing the way I *think* about what I eat, it all became so simple. I've ditched the 'old me' notions of which food goes with what, that bolognese sauce goes with spaghetti, roast beef goes with roast potatoes, and curry goes with rice. And guess what? I don't miss any of it.

I thoroughly enjoy the food I eat. I'm never hungry. I don't hanker for carbohydrates. Everything seems to taste more – bigger, better, tastier.

I've been eating this way for three years now. I'm tweaking, adapting and evolving my recipes all the time, and I've even started to have a go at proper, luxurious desserts (see pages 240–53), using sugar replacements.

This is not a 'diet', as such. It's just the way I eat now, a formula I have evolved from reading and researching all kinds of other eating regimes, which has worked for me. It's a cross-breed, a mix or mongrel that I've honed to make my own. I haven't sacrificed flavour or pleasure and I've lost 11 stone.

When I get up, I need some protein to keep me going through what is pretty much always a busy day. I might start with yoghurt, a quick omelette or even a cooked breakfast (see page 93). For lunch, I'll often have a big salad with lots of meat and veg, or perhaps a hearty broth. In the evening I sometimes cook one of my favourite minced meat dishes, braises or roasts, often making more than I need so I have the start of a tasty lunch the next day too. Or, depending on what I've eaten earlier in the day, it may be a substantial soup, hot salad or sustaining omelette.

I've found this way of eating easy to integrate into my life. The recipes are tasty and filling, so you can share them with your family and friends without them knowing that they're eating 'diet food' and without you feeling isolated.

USING THIS BOOK
While I didn't want to get hung up with calorie counts and grams of fat when I was putting together this book – it's just not that kind of diet – I do include net carb counts at the end of each recipe. Decreasing carbs lowers your body's blood sugar levels. This causes the body to burn stored fat for energy, which ultimately leads to weight loss. The 'net' carb count is just the total

carbohydrate count that a serving of food contains after you've deducted the fibre content and any sugar alcohols – in other words the net carb value has a significant impact on your blood sugar levels.

Carbohydrates are often referred to as 'bad' or 'good', 'simple' or 'complex', 'high GI' or 'low GI'. It can be confusing, but essentially, when we eat carbs they are broken down into glucose for energy and then absorbed into the bloodstream, raising blood sugar levels. But not all carbs are equal. The fibre content of carb foods affects the rate of absorption of the glucose and the impact it has on blood sugar levels. A high-fibre carbohydrate has less effect on your weight than a low-fibre carb. High-fibre carbs are complex carbs, with a low GI. Low-fibre carbs are simple and have a high GI.

A low-carb diet is classified as one with a carbohydrate intake of less than 100g per day, though this varies somewhat, depending on body size and activity levels. As carbohydrates are the body's preferred energy choice, when carbohydrate intake is low, the body switches to utilising fat and protein instead. I try to stay below 90g of carbohydrate per day. The recipe portions here are me-size – designed to satisfy a hungry bloke who is on his feet and on the go all of the time. If your lifestyle is a bit more sedentary, adjust the portion size down a little. You should never feel hungry, but you shouldn't feel stuffed either.

While some of the recipes in this book require slow cooking, lots of them can be assembled pretty quickly. If you're searching for an idea for a quick lunch or dinner, look out for ⏱.

When you're on a low-carb diet, one of the biggest challenges can be to try and work out what to have for lunch that isn't a sandwich. The recipes in the book that are really good for cooking in advance and putting into a lunchbox are signalled with 💼.

If you are going to follow my plan, you need to have willpower. It won't be easy because you need to break old habits and learn new ones, but I promise it's worth it. Once you get stuck in, you'll never look back.

STORE CUPBOARD

If you rummaged around in my cupboards at home, these are some of the ingredients you'd find. Not all of them promote the release of dopamine, but they do add flavour, depth and texture to my meals.

Anchovies Salted anchovies preserved in oil are one of the most versatile ingredients around. You can add them whole to salads, mash them into rubs for roast meat or whiz them up in dressings.

Bisto gravy granules Don't laugh! I use them a lot to add depth of flavour and richness to sauces in casseroles. It helps thicken them too.

Coconut flour This is a high-fibre, gluten-free flour which has a low GI and so doesn't cause a spike in blood sugar levels. It can be used to thicken sauces and in crispy coatings, and as a substitute for wheat flour in some recipes.

Dried herbs Not all herbs work well when dried, but I often use a good sprinkle of *herbes de Provence* in rich casseroles.

Dried mushrooms Rich in umami flavour, I use these whole to lend their flavour and meaty texture to soups and stews. I also blitz them in a small food processor to make mushroom powder, which I use as a seasoning.

Dried seaweed This is widely available now (even from supermarkets) and it's such a brilliant ingredient for adding deep, salty flavour. Try adding it to clear broths or even shredding and adding it to simple omelettes.

Gherkins or cornichons These are great for adding crunch to salads.

Mustard I keep jars of English and Dijon mustards, to add flavour and heat to marinades and dressings.

Nuts and seeds I use nuts such as pecans, almonds, hazelnuts and walnuts to add crunch to salads and to finish soups. I like sesame seeds too.

Pickled green chillies These are lovely served as they are with grilled meats, or chopped up in salads to add a bit of heat.

Pork scratchings I'm only half joking when I say I'm not sure I could have got through this without them! They're a great snack, but also I use them quite a lot in cooking to create savoury crumble toppings and crunchy coatings.

Soy sauce I use soy sauce all the time, both as a condiment but also in dressings and marinades.

Spices It's a good idea to have a decent range at your disposal. These are the ones I use all of the time: cayenne pepper, chilli powder, ground cumin, cumin seeds, ground coriander, coriander seeds, curry powder, yellow mustard seeds and smoked paprika.

Sriracha sauce This is very useful when you want to add instant heat to dressings and marinades. Try squeezing a bit over omelettes too.

Stock cubes One of the best short cuts around, I use these all the time.

Sugar replacements I use erythritol and sometimes inulin (brilliant for caramelising) as sugar replacements in this book.

Tabasco sauce The best thing to reach for when you want to add some instant fire to a dish.

Tinned consommé I always have a few tins in the cupboard, as it's often just the thing you need to enrich soups and stews.

Tinned fish Oily fish such as tuna or sardines are very good when you want to rustle up a quick, nutritious lunch.

Vinegars Red, white, cider and malt, they all have their place to sharpen up sauces or marinades.

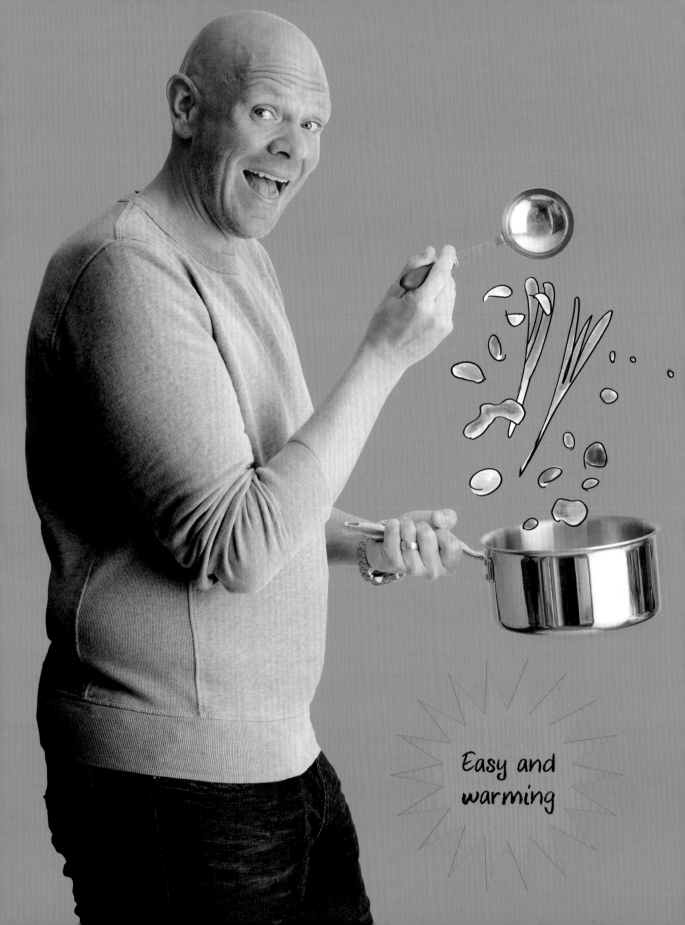

Easy and warming

SOUPS & BROTHS

MY NEW WAY OF EATING has taught me to appreciate just how versatile and infinitely adaptable soups and broths are. These days, when I'm looking for something simple and satisfying, they are among the first recipes I turn to.

Whether you want something light and fresh, such as mushroom and asparagus broth (page 30), or something rich and creamy, like curried cauliflower soup (page 32), you'll find a soup or broth in this chapter to suit your appetite and mood. Most of the recipes are very easy to make and I hope many of them will soon become firm favourites.

When we think of traditionally satisfying soups, they tend to be quite thick because we use potatoes, flour or other high-carb ingredients to give them body. Some of the soups here are, by necessity, thinner and lighter, but I hope you'll agree they're none the worse for that.

When I was creating these recipes, I was constantly trying to work out how to add different layers of flavour and texture so that you'd never miss the comforting mouthfeel of, say a classic vichyssoise or a carrot and coriander soup. I hope I've succeeded by exploiting soup's infinite capacity to carry flavour, whether you are looking for something quite delicate or craving a soup packed with spices.

The recipes are flexible and endlessly adaptable, so use them as a starting point – a foundation on which you can build your own customised soup. If you've got some slow-cooked pork belly left over from dinner, add it to the courgette noodle and salami soup (page 49), instead of, or as well as, the salami. Don't care for duck? Use leftover roast chicken in the slow-cooked duck and red cabbage broth (page 44) instead.

All of these soups can make a nice, satisfying main course all on their own – just ladle them into a big bowl and tuck in. They're also brilliant when you're facing that other dieting dilemma: what do you take to work for your packed lunch when you can't have a sandwich? If you've got a good, wide-mouthed thermos, most of these soups would travel well and keep you satisfied and full of energy all afternoon.

Wherever possible, I've used feel-good, dopamine-enhancing ingredients such as the leafy greens in the spinach, bacon and mint soup (page 52) and pak choi in the fiery squid soup (page 39). And of course, I've added my favourite mood-boosting chillies wherever I can.

One of the challenges I faced when it came to creating soups and broths for my new low-carb approach to eating, was the accompaniments and finishing touches. Could a bowl of soup really be just as good without bread or croûtons? I had to think creatively to come up with alternatives. Now I use pork scratchings, crisp-fried bacon pieces or Parmesan crisps (page 34) in place of croûtons. Or I add lightly cooked vegetables at the last minute for a nice textural bite, as for the Polish sausage, cabbage and cheese soup (page 57).

One of the final things I came to appreciate about soups and broths is that you can't eat them quickly. You have to slow down, which has always been a bit of a challenge for me! When you read traditional diet books, they often tell you to eat slowly and savour every bite and I never really got it before. I understand it better now. Taking a slower pace, enjoying each mouthful, gives your brain a chance to catch up with your belly so you can stop once you feel full, which is a great habit to get into.

Finishing touches

These are some of my favourite soup toppings:
* Pork scratchings
* Crisp-fried bacon pieces
* Dopamine-rich toasted nuts and seeds (page 61)
* Snippets of seaweed, wilted into the hot broth at the last minute (a great source of tyrosine)
* Crisp-fried bits of fish or squid
* Parmesan crisps (page 34)
* Diced salami

Light mushroom and asparagus broth

Packed full of umami – the rich, satisfying savoury flavour that mushrooms are so full of – this is incredibly tasty. It can be easily adapted too: swap garlic and parsley for other herbs, or even seaweed if you like. Or, for a more substantial dish, stir in some leftover roast chicken or pork.

Serves: 4

Carb count: 27g per person

2 chicken stock cubes
60g dried mixed mushrooms
4 tbsp chopped flat-leaf parsley
    (stalks saved and tied together
    with kitchen string)
3 tbsp clear honey
70ml dark soy sauce
200ml white wine
300g portobello mushrooms, diced
1 onion, halved and thinly sliced
A bunch of asparagus (about
    350g), stems peeled, chopped
    into 1–2cm pieces
150g button mushrooms, sliced
2 tbsp vegetable oil
8 garlic cloves, grated
Sea salt and freshly ground black
    pepper

① Bring 800ml water to the boil in a large pan. Crumble in the stock cubes and whisk until dissolved. Take off the heat and add the dried mushrooms and bundle of parsley stalks. Leave to stand for about 20 minutes.

② In a separate large saucepan (one that has a light-coloured interior so you will be able to see the colour of the caramel), warm the honey over a medium heat, stirring, until it begins to bubble. Stop stirring and cook, watching it carefully, to a rich, golden brown caramel. Immediately pour on the soy sauce, which will stop the cooking, then add the wine.

③ Scoop out the soaked mushrooms and parsley stalks from the stock and add them to the soy mixture. Pour the stock through a muslin-lined sieve into the pan – this will help to remove any grit from the dried mushrooms.

④ Bring the broth to a steady simmer. Add the portobello mushrooms and onion and cook for 3–4 minutes. Add the asparagus and poach for 2 minutes. Stir in the button mushrooms.

⑤ Heat the oil in a frying pan over a high heat. Add the garlic and cook, stirring until lightly browned; don't let it burn. Remove the bundle of parsley stalks from the soup and then stir in the fried garlic and chopped parsley. Serve immediately, in warmed bowls.

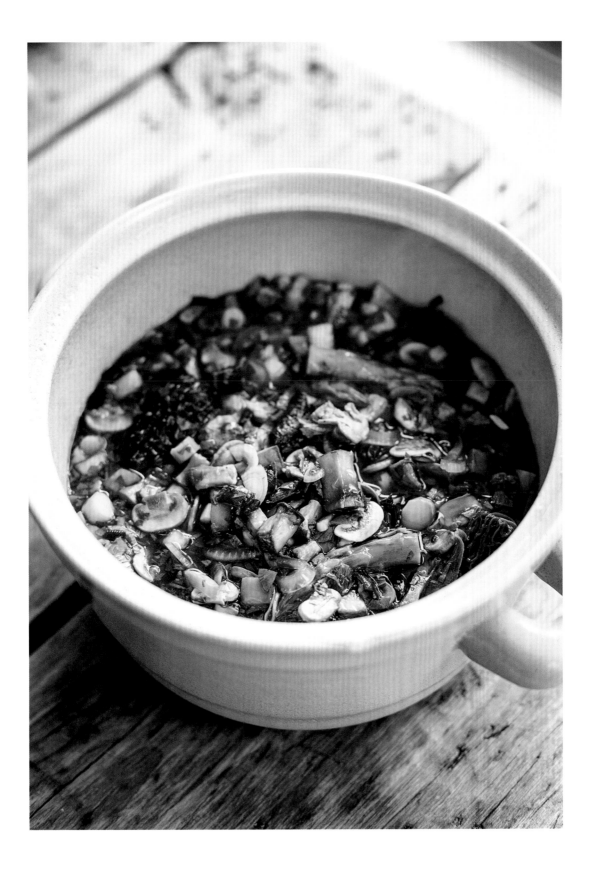

Curried cauliflower soup

I've eaten a lot of cauliflower on my low-carb diet and I've grown to love it. When it's cooked and puréed like this, it takes on such a rich, creamy texture that it feels quite indulgent, particularly when combined with the coconut and cream cheese. It takes on spices beautifully, too.

Serves: 4
Carb count: 22g per person

50g dried onion flakes
2 tbsp vegetable oil
50g butter
1 onion, diced
2 garlic cloves, grated
1½ tbsp curry powder
1 chicken or vegetable stock cube
1 large cauliflower (about 800g), broken into florets
200ml coconut cream
200g cream cheese
4 tbsp chopped coriander, tender stems and all
2 hot green chillies, sliced, seeds and all
Finely grated zest of 1 lime
Sea salt and cayenne pepper

1. Preheat the oven to 180°C/Fan 160°C/Gas 4. Scatter the onion flakes on a baking tray, trickle on the oil, give it a stir and season with salt. Bake for 5 minutes, or until the onion flakes are golden brown. Set aside to cool.

2. In a large saucepan, melt the butter over a medium-low heat. Add the onion and garlic and sweat gently, stirring from time to time, for 10–15 minutes until soft. Sprinkle on the curry powder and cook, stirring, for 2–3 minutes.

3. Now pour in 1 litre water and crumble in the stock cube. Bring to the boil and add the cauliflower florets. Turn the heat down to a simmer and cook for 5–10 minutes, until the cauliflower is soft.

4. Stir in the coconut cream and cream cheese until fully combined. Bring back to the boil then take the pan off the heat.

5. Blitz with a stick blender, or in a jug blender or food processor. If you've time, pass the soup through a sieve into a clean pan at this point – this will give the soup an unbelievably silky and delicious texture. Warm gently and season to taste with salt and cayenne pepper.

6. Ladle the soup into warmed bowls and scatter over the toasted onion flakes, coriander, chilli and lime zest.

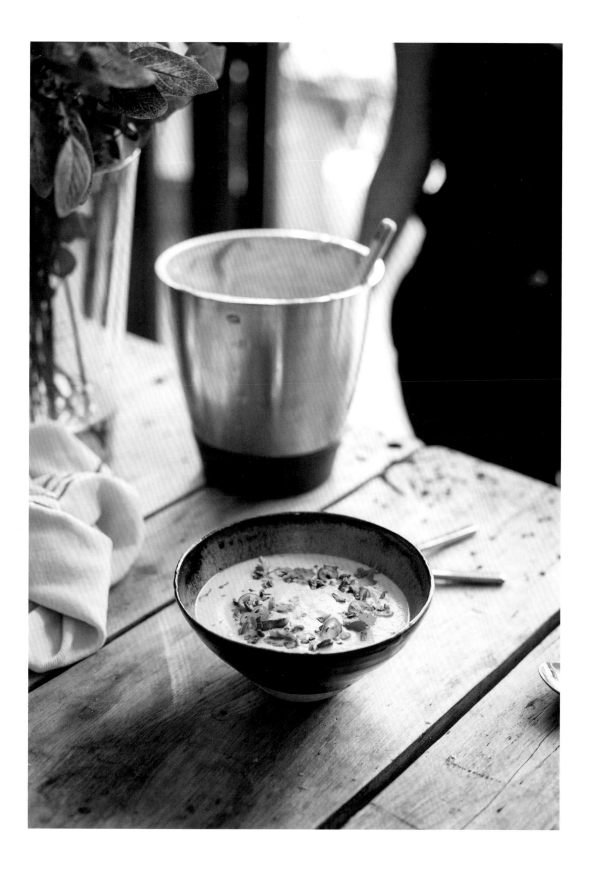

Bouillabaisse with Parmesan crisps

Full of great flavours, bouillabaisse is one of the world's finest soups. I'm not going to lie, it does take a bit of preparation and patience, but none of it is difficult and you can do a lot ahead if you like. It really is worth the effort.

Serves: 4–6

Carb count: 23–15g per person

For the bouillabaisse:
500g fish bones, rinsed (ask your fishmonger for these)
1 red mullet (500g or larger), cleaned and scaled, roughly cut into 10cm chunks
3 celery sticks, roughly chopped
1 onion, roughly chopped
1 carrot, roughly chopped
4 garlic cloves, peeled
2 star anise
½ tbsp white peppercorns
½ tbsp fennel seeds
1 tbsp tomato purée
400g tin chopped tomatoes
3–4 tbsp brandy
3–4 tbsp pastis, such as Pernod
3–4 tbsp vermouth
A large pinch of saffron strands
1 litre fish stock or light chicken stock
Finely pared zest and juice of 1 orange
Finely pared zest and juice of 1 lemon
Sea salt and freshly ground black or white pepper

1 Preheat the oven to 180°C/Fan 160°C/ Gas 4. Put the fish bones and red mullet pieces into a roasting tin. Put the chopped vegetables and garlic into a separate roasting tin. Place both tins in the oven. Roast for 20 minutes, until the red mullet is cooked through and the fish bones are browned, then remove from the oven. Continue to roast the vegetables for a further 10 minutes until browned around the edges.

2 Tip the bones and fish into a large saucepan and add the roasted vegetables, star anise, white peppercorns, fennel seeds and tomato purée. Cook, stirring, over a medium heat for 15 minutes.

3 Add the tomatoes, alcohol and saffron, along with the stock and 2 litres water. Bring to the boil then turn down the heat and simmer gently for 25–30 minutes. Remove from the heat and leave to cool slightly for 10 minutes.

4 Pass the soup through a fine sieve into a clean pan, pressing down to extract as much flavour as possible. Add the citrus zests and juices. Return to the heat and simmer until reduced by half. Season well with salt and pepper, then pass through a muslin-lined sieve into a clean pan. (At this stage, you can cool the soup and keep it covered in the fridge for 2–3 days.)

For the rouille:
2 free-range egg yolks
2 tbsp Dijon mustard
2 tbsp chopped, jarred roasted
    red peppers
Juice of ½ lemon
1 tbsp white wine vinegar
1 tsp smoked paprika
4 garlic cloves, grated
1 small red chilli, finely chopped,
    seeds and all
A small pinch of saffron strands
200ml good-quality extra virgin
    olive oil

For the Parmesan crisps:
70g Parmesan cheese, freshly
    finely grated

⑤ To make the rouille, put all the ingredients except the oil into a blender or food processor and blitz until smooth. With the motor running, slowly add the olive oil in a thin stream until the mixture thickens and emulsifies. Season, cover and refrigerate if not using immediately.

⑥ For the Parmesan crisps, preheat the oven to 180°C/Fan 160°C/ Gas 4. Line a baking sheet with a non-stick silicone mat or baking parchment. Sprinkle on the cheese and bake until it melts and starts to turn golden, about 6–8 minutes. Leave to cool, then break into rough pieces or shards.

⑦ Gently heat the soup and divide between warmed bowls. Top with the Parmesan crisps and finish with a dollop of rouille.

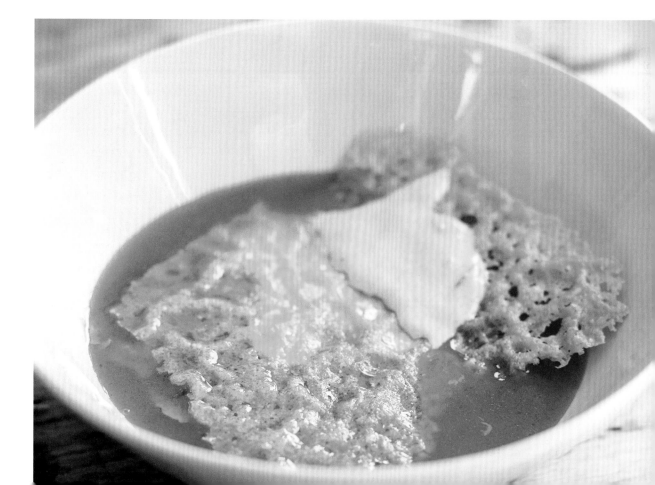

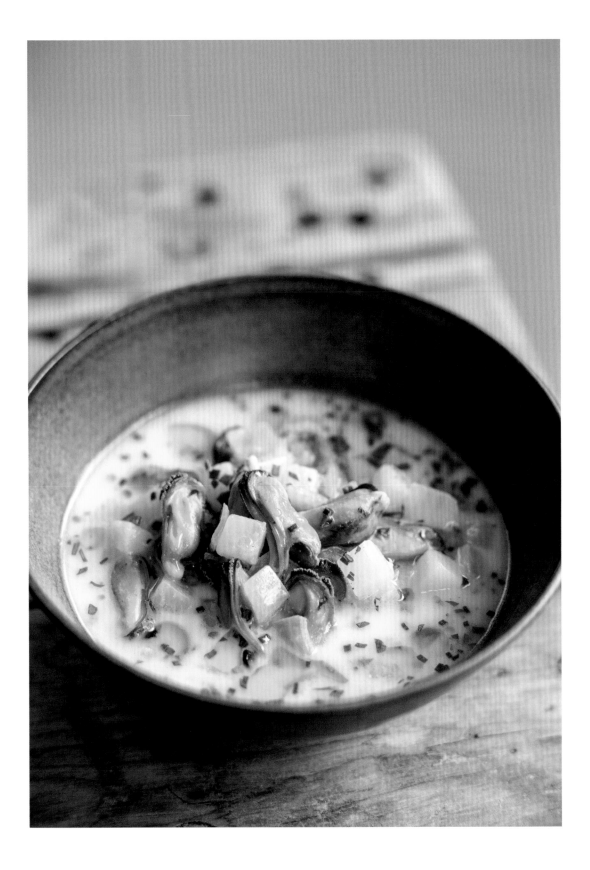

Rich mussel broth

This is a soupy version of *moules marinières*, full of flavour and just perfect for a light evening meal. It takes a little time to clean the mussels and remove them from their shells, but I promise you it's worth it.

Serves: 4

Carb count: 20g per person

2kg fresh mussels in their shells
1 chicken stock cube
75g butter, diced
1 large onion, diced
150g turnip, peeled and cut into
    1cm dice
150g kohlrabi, peeled and cut
    into 1cm dice
4 tbsp crème fraîche
2 tbsp chopped parsley leaves
2 tbsp chopped chives
Freshly ground black pepper
Good-quality extra virgin olive oil,
    to finish

1. First clean the mussels. Discard any with broken shells and any that do not close when you tap them firmly. Pull away the beards. Rinse the mussels thoroughly under cold water.

2. Pour 350ml water into a small saucepan, then crumble in the stock cube and bring to the boil.

3. Warm up a large pan that has a tight-fitting lid over a high heat. Tip in the mussels, pour on the hot stock and cover with the lid. Cook for 3–5 minutes until the shells open.

4. Tip the mussels and liquor into a muslin-lined colander placed over a bowl to strain the stock into the bowl. Pick the mussels out of their shells and set aside; discard any that remain closed. Reserve the stock.

5. In a large saucepan over a medium-low heat, melt the butter and heat until it stops foaming. Add the onion, turnip and kohlrabi and sauté until soft, stirring from time to time, about 10–15 minutes.

6. Pour in the stock, bring to the boil and simmer until reduced by half. Stir in the crème fraîche then add the mussels and season with pepper to taste – it shouldn't need salt as the mussels and stock are quite salty. Ladle into warmed bowls, scatter over the herbs and finish with a trickle of olive oil.

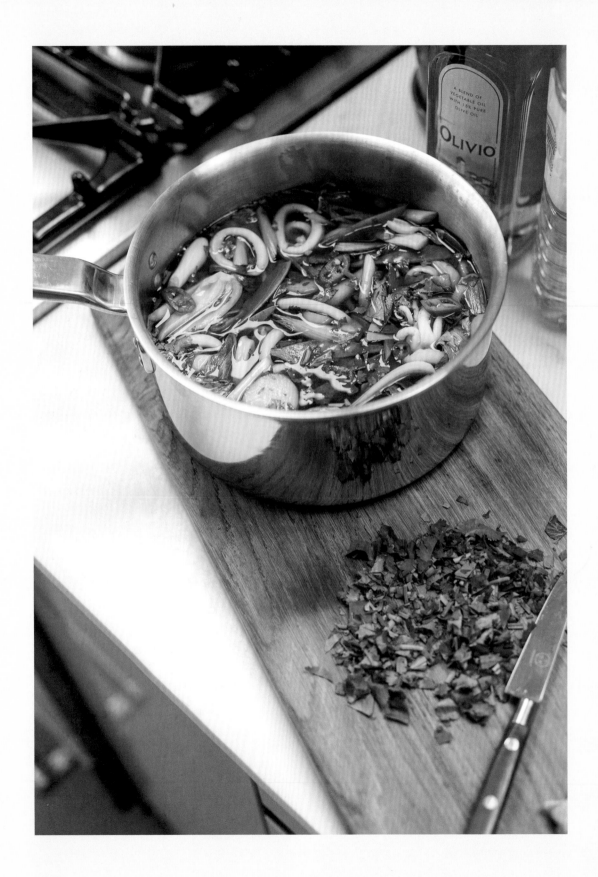

Fiery squid soup

This isn't an authentic broth from any particular part of Asia but it has all the huge Asian flavours that I love so much. It's fresh and warming, and leaves you feeling satisfied and ready to go!

Serves: 4

Carb count: 27g per person

3 tbsp clear honey
100ml dark soy sauce
2 chicken stock cubes
4 garlic cloves, thinly sliced
5cm knob of fresh ginger, grated
330g fresh squid, with tentacles, cleaned and rinsed
4 pak choi, roughly chopped
225g tin water chestnuts, drained and halved
100g mangetout, halved
A bunch of spring onions, trimmed and cut into 2cm pieces
½ bunch of coriander, chopped, tender stems and all
3 red chillies, sliced, seeds and all
Juice of 1–2 limes, to taste

① In a large pan (one with a light-coloured interior so you will be able to see the colour of the caramel), warm the honey over a medium heat, stirring, until it begins to bubble. Stop stirring and cook to a rich, golden brown caramel – keep an eye on it, as you don't want it to scorch. As soon as it reaches the right colour, pour in the soy sauce; this will stop the cooking.

② Pour in 1 litre water and then crumble in the stock cubes. Bring to a simmer and add the garlic and ginger. Let the broth simmer for a further minute.

③ Meanwhile, cut the squid into 1cm rings and roughly chop the tentacles.

④ Add the squid to the broth together with all the remaining ingredients. Give it a stir and simmer very gently for a minute, just to warm the squid through – any longer and it will become tough. Serve the soup immediately, in warmed bowls.

Crispy squid and seaweed soup

This soup has a distinct and delicious flavour of the sea, which comes from the tasty seaweed (available from health food shops, some supermarkets and online). One of my favourite inventions in my quest to be low-carb is the crispy squid coating. A crunchy combination of coconut flour and crushed pork scratchings, it's great on all kinds of fish.

Serves: 4

Carb count: 14g per person

20g dried wakame seaweed
15g dried dulse seaweed
2 tbsp white miso paste
2 tbsp dark soy sauce
2 tsp sesame oil
1 tsp freshly ground white pepper
Vegetable oil, for deep- and
    shallow-frying
200g firm tofu, drained, patted dry
    on kitchen paper and cut into
    2cm cubes
200g fresh squid, cleaned and cut
    into 1cm rings
100g samphire
A bunch of spring onions, trimmed
    and cut into 1cm pieces
4 garlic cloves, grated
1–2 red chillies, sliced, seeds
    and all

For the crispy coating:
130g pork scratchings
50g coconut flour, plus extra
    to dust
1 tsp cracked black pepper
1 tsp sea salt
4 free-range egg yolks
100ml milk

1. Put the wakame and dulse seaweeds into a bowl, pour on 600ml warm water and leave to soak for 20 minutes. Strain the liquor through a fine sieve into a clean pan and add another 600ml water. Reserve the seaweed.

2. Whisk the miso paste into the liquor and bring to a simmer. Add the soy sauce, sesame oil and white pepper, then the reserved seaweed. Simmer for 10–15 minutes.

3. Meanwhile, heat a thin layer of oil in a non-stick frying pan over a high heat. Add the tofu and cook, turning gently as necessary, until lightly toasted on all sides. Carefully remove with a spatula and drain on kitchen paper.

4. For the coating, crush the pork scratchings in their bags with a rolling pin, then open the bags and tip the crumbs into a bowl. Add the coconut flour, cracked black pepper and salt; mix well. In another bowl, beat the egg yolks with the milk. Put some coconut flour into a third bowl.

5. To coat the squid pieces, dip them a few at a time into the coconut flour, shake off any excess, then dip them into the egg mix, and finally into the crumb mix, making sure they are well coated all over.

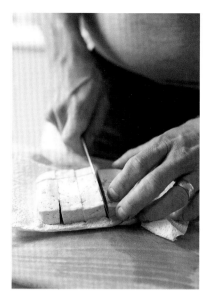

6. Heat the oil in a deep-fryer or other deep, heavy-bottomed pan to 180°C; the pan must be no more than one-third full. Check the temperature with a cook's thermometer.

7. Fry the squid rings in batches until golden and crisp, about 3 minutes; don't overcrowd the pan. Drain the squid on kitchen paper.

8. Add the samphire, spring onions, garlic and chillies to the soup then gently stir in the tofu. Serve in warmed bowls, with the crispy squid heaped on the top.

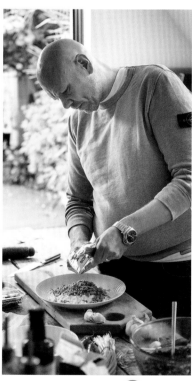

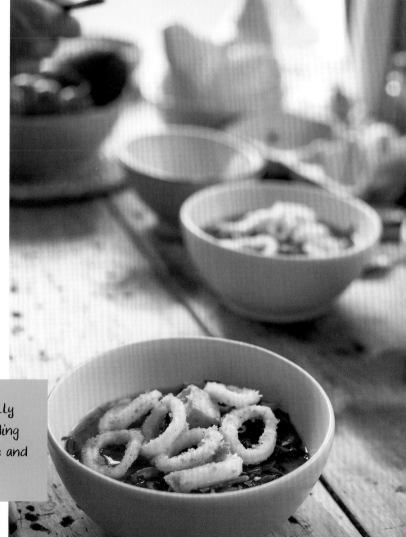

The Dope: Seaweeds add a really great depth of flavour – try adding some to all kinds of clear broths and you'll see what I mean.

Pulled chicken and shiitake mushroom broth

I love this easy and incredibly tasty soup. It takes a little time to prepare, but for me it's one of those 'go to' dishes that are both healthy and hearty.

Serves: 4

Carb count: 28g per person

2 chicken stock cubes
2 lemongrass stems, bruised with the flat blade of a knife
2 lime leaves
4 free-range chicken legs
3 tbsp clear honey
3 tbsp dark soy sauce
200g shiitake mushrooms
4 celery sticks, tough strings removed, sliced
1 onion, halved and thinly sliced
2 garlic cloves, grated
2 tbsp vegetable oil
2 bunches of spring onions, trimmed and finely sliced
2 green chillies, sliced, seeds and all
2 tbsp sherry vinegar
Sea salt and freshly ground black pepper

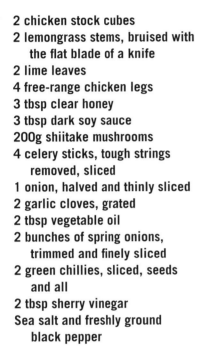

1 Pour 1.2 litres water into a large pan and crumble in the stock cubes. Bring to the boil and add the lemongrass and lime leaves. Add the chicken legs, lower the heat and simmer gently for 45–60 minutes until they are very tender. Lift out the chicken legs; let cool. Pass the stock through a fine sieve into a bowl.

2 In a separate pan (one with a light-coloured interior so you will be able to see the colour of the caramel), warm the honey over a medium heat, stirring, until it begins to bubble. Stop stirring and cook, watching carefully, to a rich, golden brown caramel. Immediately pour on the soy sauce; this will stop the cooking. Pour in the strained stock and bring to the boil.

3 Turn the heat down, add the mushrooms and celery and poach very gently for about 5 minutes until just cooked. Add the onion and garlic.

4 Using a couple of forks, pull apart and flake the meat and skin from the chicken legs. Heat the oil in a non-stick frying pan over a medium-high heat and fry half of the pulled chicken until crisp. Drain on kitchen paper and season with salt and pepper.

5 Add the remaining chicken to the broth, with the spring onions, chillies and sherry vinegar. Season with salt and pepper to taste. Add the crispy chicken and serve in warmed bowls.

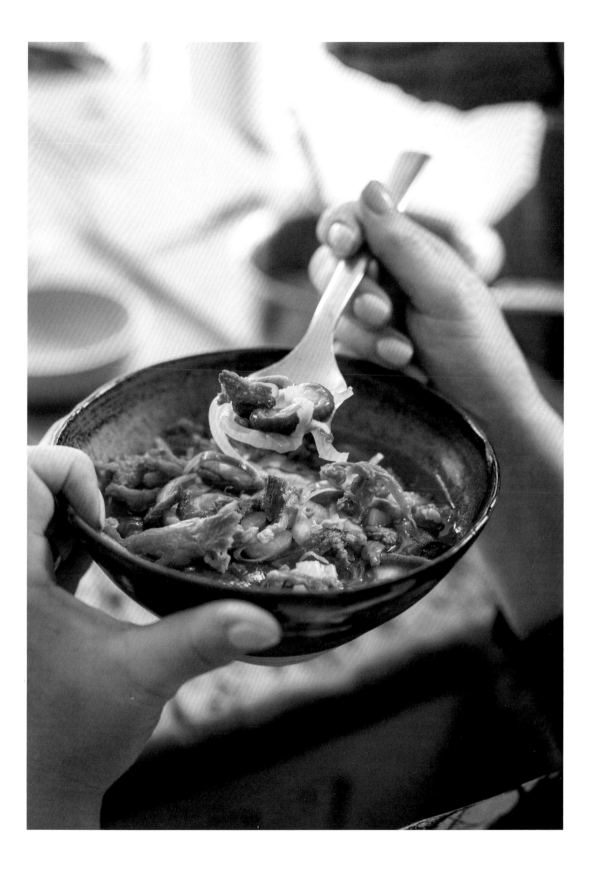

Slow-cooked duck and red cabbage broth

This soup is simple to make but it's crammed with great flavours and textures – a winning combination of crunchy, sweet and sour. If you double up the amount of duck, you can easily serve it as a tasty main course. Pour the fat rendered from the duck legs into a jar, seal and keep in the fridge – it's great for frying and roasting.

Serves: 4
Carb count: 27g per person

4 duck legs
500g red cabbage, core removed
2 onions, halved and finely sliced
1½ tbsp flaky sea salt
½ tsp black peppercorns
2 star anise
2 cloves
2 chicken stock cubes
3 tbsp clear honey
150ml brown malt vinegar
1 tbsp caraway seeds, toasted in
**   a dry frying pan until fragrant**
Finely grated zest of 1 orange
1 tbsp chopped rosemary
Sea salt and freshly ground
**   black pepper**

1 Preheat the oven to 180°C/Fan 160°C/Gas 4. Place the duck legs in a roasting tin and roast for 1 hour, then turn the oven setting down to 160°C/Fan 140°C/Gas 3 and roast for a further 1½–2 hours, until the skin is really crisp and the meat is tender.

2 In the meantime, finely shred the cabbage and place in a large bowl with the onions. Sprinkle over the flaky salt and massage it in with your hands. Mix thoroughly and leave to sit for 20 minutes. Tip the vegetables into a colander and rinse off the salt under cold running water.

3 When the duck legs are cooked, lift them out of the roasting tin and drain on kitchen paper. (Save the rendered duck fat, see above.) When cold enough to handle, shred the duck, keeping the duck skin on the meat.

4 Bring 1 litre water to the boil in a saucepan. Tie the black peppercorns, star anise and cloves in a piece of muslin with kitchen string. Add to the boiling water then crumble in the stock cubes. Lower the heat and simmer gently to infuse for 10–15 minutes.

5 In a separate large pan (with a light-coloured interior so you will be able to see the colour of the caramel), warm the honey over a medium heat, stirring, until it begins to bubble. Stop stirring and cook, watching carefully, to a rich, golden brown caramel. Immediately pour in the malt vinegar; this will stop the cooking.

⑥ Pour on the infused stock, add the cabbage and onion, stir and warm through. Remove the muslin bundle. Add the caraway seeds and season with salt and pepper if necessary.

⑦ Ladle the soup into warmed bowls and top with the shredded duck. Scatter over the orange zest and chopped rosemary to serve.

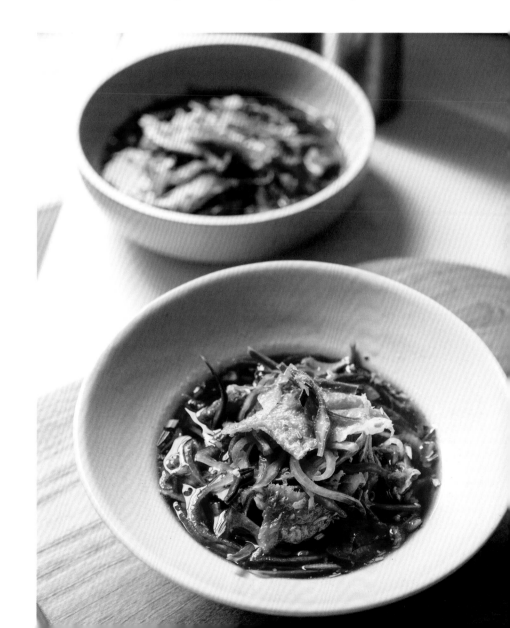

Crispy duck, coleslaw and fennel soup

This gutsy soup was an experiment that really worked – teaming up one of my favourite coleslaw combinations with some tasty shredded duck. The peppery hit you get from the cabbage and kohlrabi is really important – it gives the dish its kick.

Serves: 4

Carb count: 19g per person

1 tsp smoked paprika
½ tsp ground cinnamon
½ tsp ground cumin
½ tsp table salt
4 large duck legs
2 large carrots, coarsely grated
2 red onions, halved and thinly
    sliced
1 large white onion, halved and
    thinly sliced
1 fennel bulb, cored and thinly
    sliced
1 kohlrabi, peeled and coarsely
    grated
¼ white cabbage, cored and
    thinly sliced
½ tbsp flaky sea salt
2 chicken stock cubes
3 large, pickled green chillies,
    sliced
2 garlic cloves, grated
½ tbsp cracked black pepper
3 tbsp mayonnaise
2 tbsp English mustard
2 tbsp fennel seeds, toasted in
    a dry frying pan until fragrant
Grated zest of 1 orange
4 tbsp chopped dill
Sea salt and freshly ground
    black pepper

1 Preheat the oven to 180°C/Fan 160°C/Gas 4. Mix the smoked paprika, ground cinnamon, cumin and table salt together and rub into the duck legs. Place them in a roasting tin and roast for 1 hour.

2 Now turn the oven setting down to 160°C/Fan 140°C/Gas 3 and roast the duck legs for a further 1½–2 hours, until the skin is crisp and the meat is tender. Lift out and drain on kitchen paper. When cool enough to handle, shred into bite-sized pieces; keep warm.

3 Meanwhile, in a large bowl, toss the carrots, onions, fennel, kohlrabi and cabbage with the flaky salt and leave to soften for 20 minutes.

4 Bring 750ml water to the boil in a large saucepan, crumble in the stock cubes and whisk until dissolved.

5 Tip the vegetables into a colander and rinse off the salt under cold running water. Drain well and place in a bowl. Add the chillies, garlic and cracked pepper. Tip into the warm stock and heat up gently. Remove from the heat and stir through the mayonnaise and mustard. Taste and adjust the seasoning.

6 Ladle the soup into warmed bowls, scatter over the toasted fennel seeds, orange zest and chopped dill, then pile the crispy duck on top to serve.

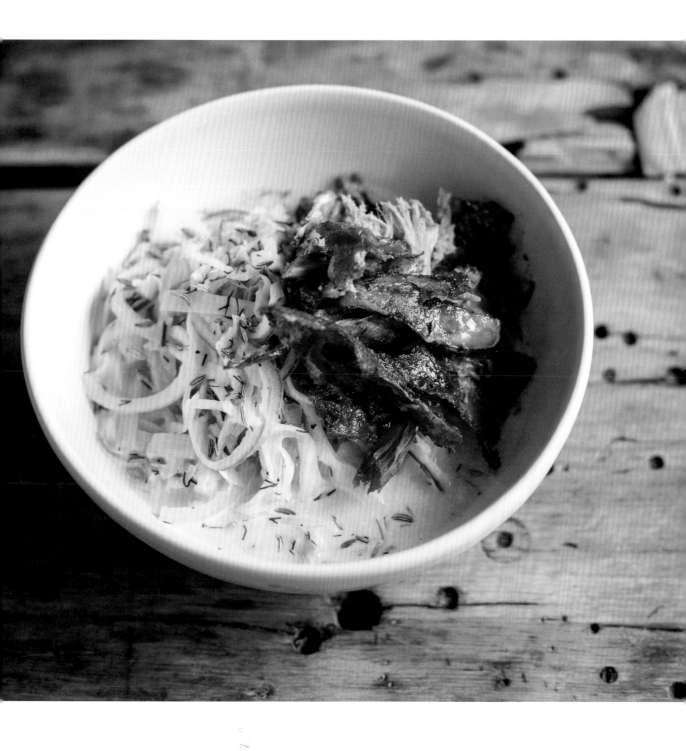

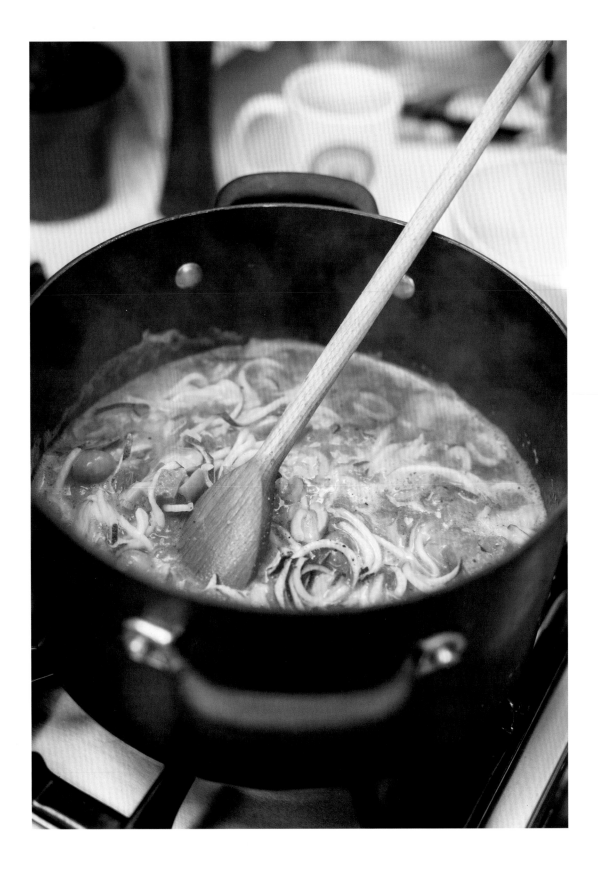

Courgette noodle and salami soup

This is a great soup if you're looking for something easy to make for a quick lunch or dinner. It has a lovely balance of salty and sour from the salami and artichokes, and the soft mozzarella makes the broth deliciously creamy. You'll need a spiralizer to turn the courgettes into noodles, but it's a good investment as it opens up all kinds of tasty, low-carb alternatives to pasta for soups and salads.

Serves: 4

Carb count: 7g per person

350g Milano salami (in one piece)
2–3 large courgettes (about 300g)
2 chicken or vegetable stock cubes
150g marinated artichokes, quartered
100g green olives, stoned and halved
2 balls of mozzarella (about 125g each), diced
A bunch of basil (about 25g), leaves picked from stems and torn
2 tbsp extra virgin olive oil
Sea salt and cracked black pepper

1 Pour 1 litre water into a saucepan and bring to the boil.

2 Meanwhile, cut the salami into 1cm dice and spiralize the courgettes into thin noodles.

3 Crumble the stock cubes into the boiling water and whisk to dissolve. Turn the heat down to a simmer and tip in the salami. Simmer for a couple of minutes.

4 Add the courgette noodles to the pan, along with the artichokes and olives, and warm through for 1–2 minutes.

5 Stir in the diced mozzarella and torn basil leaves and season with salt and cracked black pepper to taste.

6 Drizzle with olive oil and serve the soup immediately, in warmed bowls – it's important not to let the courgette noodles overcook.

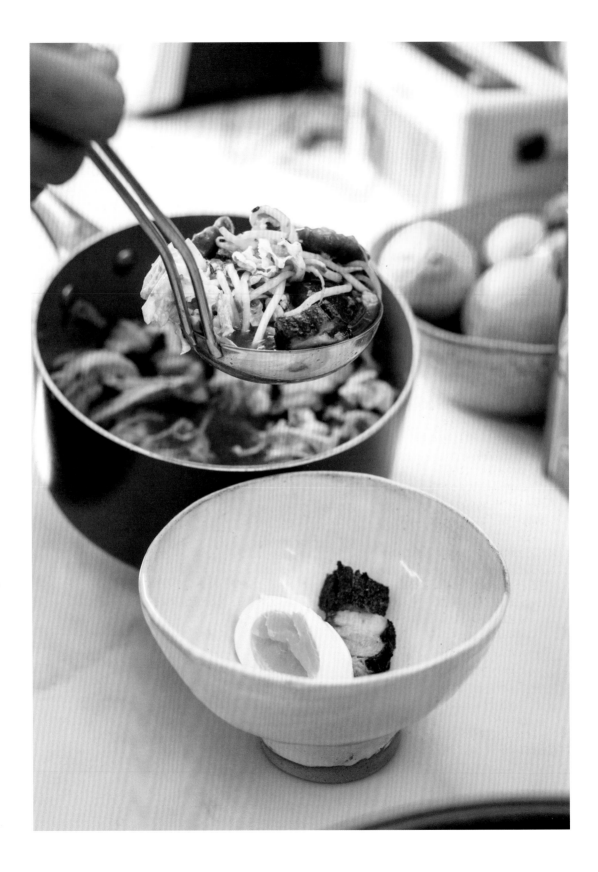

Spicy, porky lettuce soup

This soup is a mixture of great textures, from soft, chewy shiitake mushrooms to crispy pork belly and crunchy Chinese lettuce. It's brilliantly aromatic too. Feel free to make it as hot and spicy as you want. Remember, the hotter it is, the better it is for your endorphin release!

Serves: 4

Carb count: 28g per person

2 tbsp Chinese five-spice powder
1 tbsp vegetable oil
400g pork belly, skin on, scored
2 large free-range eggs
4 red chillies, chopped, seeds and all
2 garlic cloves, grated
1 banana shallot, finely diced
5cm knob of fresh ginger, grated
2 tsp demerara sugar
2 tbsp rice wine vinegar
Juice of 1 lime
1 tsp flaky sea salt
2 chicken stock cubes
100ml dark soy sauce
1 tbsp cornflour, mixed to a paste with 2 tbsp water
200g shiitake mushrooms
A bunch of spring onions, trimmed then cut into 2cm pieces
½ bunch of mint (about 10g), leaves picked from stems and roughly torn
½ bunch of coriander (about 10g), roughly chopped, tender stems and all
½ Chinese leaf lettuce, roughly shredded
150g bean sprouts
Sea salt

1. Preheat the oven to 160°C/Fan 140°C/Gas 3. Mix the five-spice powder and oil to a paste. Rub this paste into the pork belly, season with salt and place in a roasting tin. Cook for 2½ hours until the skin is crisp and the meat tender. Set aside.

2. Bring a pan of water to the boil, add the eggs and simmer for 7 minutes, then remove from the pan and cool under cold running water.

3. Using a pestle and mortar or a mini food processor, grind the chillies, garlic, shallot, ginger and sugar to a paste. Add the rice wine vinegar, lime juice and flaky salt. Set aside.

4. In a large pan, bring 1 litre water to the boil and crumble in the stock cubes. Add the soy sauce and cornflour paste. Whisk until the stock thickens slightly, then lower the heat and whisk in the chilli mixture. Simmer for 2–3 minutes.

5. Add the shiitake mushrooms and cook for a further 2–3 minutes. Meanwhile, cut the pork into bite-sized chunks. Add to the soup with the spring onions, mint and coriander. Stir in the shredded Chinese leaf and bean sprouts.

6. Peel and halve the boiled eggs and place one half in each warmed bowl. Ladle the broth over the eggs and serve immediately.

Spinach, bacon and mint soup

This is a vibrant, rich and tasty soup. It looks healthy – which it is – but tastes really luxurious. The salty bacon goes so well with the spinach and fresh mint.

Serves: 4

Carb count: 10g per person

500g spinach leaves, tough stalks removed, or baby spinach
50g butter
250g pancetta or bacon, derinded and diced
2 onions, diced
2 garlic cloves, grated
2 chicken stock cubes
A large bunch of mint (about 25g), tough stems removed and discarded, plus a few sprigs to garnish
150g soured cream
Freshly grated nutmeg
Sea salt and freshly ground black pepper
Extra virgin olive oil, to finish

① Fill a large bowl with iced water. Bring a large pan of water to the boil and add salt. Blanch the spinach in the boiling water, just until wilted. Drain, refresh in the iced water and drain well. Squeeze out excess water in a clean tea towel.

② Melt the butter in a large saucepan over a medium-high heat. Add the pancetta and cook until crisp. Remove from the pan with a slotted spoon and drain on kitchen paper. Set aside.

③ Add the onions to the pan and sweat over a medium-low heat, stirring regularly, until soft, about 10–15 minutes. Add the garlic and stir for a minute or two. Crumble in the stock cubes, pour in 1 litre water and bring to the boil.

④ Put half of the cooked spinach into a jug blender with half of the mint and 50g of the soured cream. Add half the stock and onion mixture and blend until very smooth.

⑤ Unless serving right away, pass through a sieve into a large bowl containing two freezer blocks – to cool the soup quickly and keep its colour. Repeat with the rest of the spinach and mint, another 50g cream and remaining stock mix.

⑥ To serve, gently warm the soup in a pan; don't let it boil. Season with salt, pepper and nutmeg to taste. Pour into warmed bowls and top with the crispy pancetta and mint. Finish with the remaining soured cream and a little olive oil.

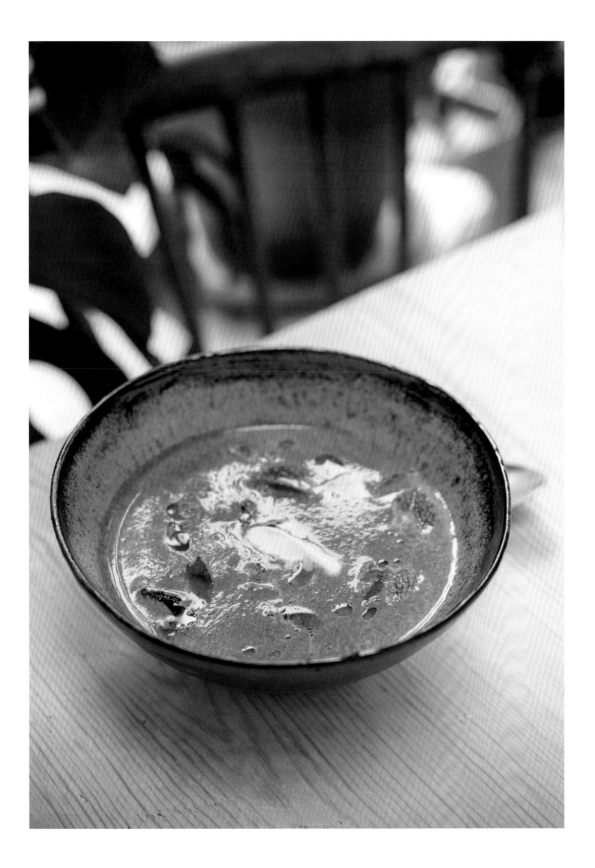

Hot pastrami and pickle broth

This is a fantastic last-minute lunch dish, which uses some of my favourite store cupboard ingredients. It's a sort of riff on a classic, American pastrami sandwich, without the bread, of course. Toasted walnuts lend a unique texture and flavour.

Serves: 4

Carb count: 20g per person

150g shelled walnuts
75g butter
2 onions, diced
150g celeriac
150g turnip
150g kohlrabi
2 chicken stock cubes
400g pastrami, diced
150g dill pickles, drained and diced, plus 150ml juice from the jar
2 large, green pickled chillies, diced
2 tbsp American-style mustard
1 tbsp cracked black pepper
4 tbsp chopped dill
Sea salt

1 Preheat the oven to 180°C/160°C/Gas 4. Scatter the walnuts on a baking tray and toast in the oven for 5–10 minutes until golden brown and fragrant. Tip onto a board and leave to cool slightly, then chop roughly.

2 In a large saucepan, melt the butter over a medium heat. When it's stopped foaming, add the onions and sauté, stirring from time to time, until soft, about 10–15 minutes.

3 Meanwhile, peel the celeriac, turnip and kohlrabi and cut into 1cm dice. Add the celeriac to the pan and cook for 3–4 minutes. Add the diced turnip and kohlrabi and sweat, stirring, for 1–2 minutes.

4 Pour in 650ml water and crumble in the stock cubes. Bring to a simmer.

5 Add the pastrami, pickles and pickle juice and cook for 1–2 minutes. Stir in the chillies, mustard and cracked black pepper. Season with salt to taste.

6 Finally, stir in the chopped toasted walnuts and chopped dill. Serve in warmed bowls.

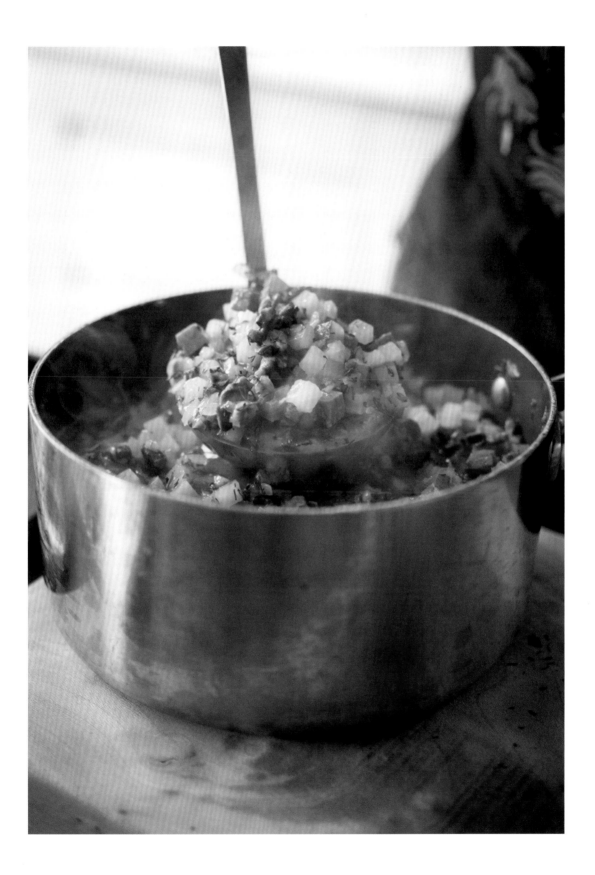

The Dope: Adding a handful of grated full-flavoured <u>cheese</u> to a bowl of soup makes it more of a substantial, main-course event.

Polish sausage, cabbage and cheese soup

This is a big, bold soup, full of hearty, strong flavours. It's just the thing for a cold winter's day, or any day when you're craving something substantial to eat. If you're able to track down some proper Polish sausage, from a Polish deli or supermarket perhaps, it will make all the difference to the flavour.

Serves: 4–6

Carb count: 14–10g per person

½ white cabbage, cored
3 tbsp freshly grated horseradish
2 tsp flaky sea salt
1 tbsp cumin seeds
1 tbsp cracked black pepper
1 tbsp curry powder
1 tsp paprika
3 tbsp olive oil
2 onions, halved and thinly sliced
3 garlic cloves, grated
2 chicken stock cubes
500g Polish kielbasa sausage, cut into 2cm chunks
150g kale, tough stems removed, roughly chopped
2 tbsp thyme leaves
3–4 tbsp brown malt vinegar
150g strong Cheddar cheese, grated
Sea salt and freshly ground black pepper

1 Finely shred the cabbage and place in a large bowl. Add the horseradish, salt, cumin, black pepper, curry powder and paprika, toss to mix and leave the cabbage to infuse and soften for 15–20 minutes.

2 In a large saucepan, warm the olive oil over a medium-low heat. Add the onions and garlic and sweat gently, stirring from time to time, until softened, about 10–15 minutes. Pour in 1 litre water and crumble in the stock cubes. Bring to the boil.

3 Add the Polish sausage and turn the heat down to a simmer. Drain the wilted cabbage then stir into the broth. Warm through for 3–5 minutes.

4 Add the kale and thyme leaves. Season with vinegar, salt and pepper to taste, then ladle into warmed bowls. Scatter over the grated cheese and serve immediately.

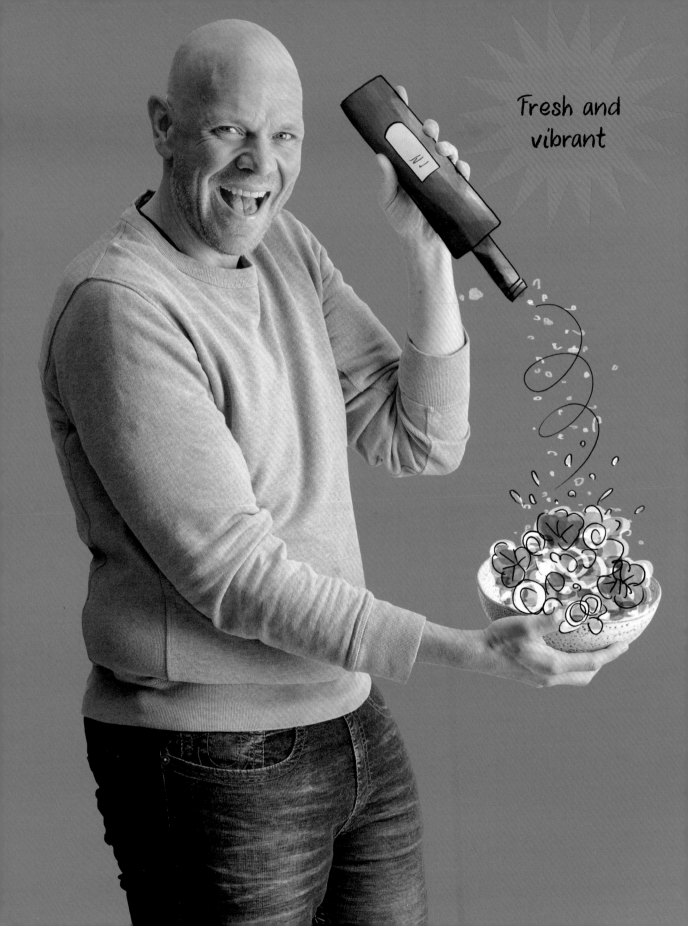

Fresh and
vibrant

HOT & COLD SALADS

BURSTING WITH DEEP FLAVOURS, vibrant colours and satisfying textures, these recipes are as far removed from a limp lettuce leaf and a slice of flavourless tomato as it's possible to get. They're some of my favourite recipes in the whole book.

Salads have always suffered a bit from being regarded as the goody-two-shoes 'healthy option' on the menu, for which you can read the 'boring option'. But nothing could be further from the truth. If you stop looking at them as part of a low-calorie or low-fat diet and start seeing them as part of a low-carb one, salads can suddenly become very exciting indeed. The salads in this chapter are some of the best things you can eat!

For me, the mighty Caesar salad is the best. It has everything: crisp Romaine lettuce leaves, a rich, creamy dressing, salty anchovies, intensely savoury cheese and the textural crunch that comes from croûtons. Most of the salads I make are built on the understanding of how those layers of flavour and texture work together. If you take a look at my mackerel, chicory and radicchio Caesar salad (page 77) and chicken, avocado and lettuce wraps (page 79), you'll get the idea. Of course, I have had to remove the carby croûton crunch, but I make up for it with the crunchy fried fish skin and crispy iceberg lettuce. Chicken and mackerel are great dopamine boosters too, and oily fish has the added benefit of being rich in Vitamin D, which is so important for healthy brain function.

I'm also a massive fan of hot salads. Wilting leaves in the pan – as in the spinach, sesame and pork scratchings salad (page 82) – gives them a silky texture and an entirely different mouthfeel, which is both satisfying and luxurious. It becomes an all-year-round salad rather than something you might eat in the garden in the summer. And, of course, popping a fried egg on top only makes it more tempting.

One of the things I realised as I created these new recipes was that when I took the heavy carb elements away from my favourite salads, I didn't miss them at all. Actually, not only did I not miss them, I realised that bland carbs had been holding my salads back over the years! Remove them, and it gives all of the other salad ingredients a chance to really shine. If you take away the potatoes from a *salade niçoise*, for example, you really start to taste the delicious olives, green beans and tomatoes.

I believe strongly in experimenting with flavours and textures and I'm always up for trying something new – to me, that's the fun part of cooking! I realise that I'm about as far away from the new tribe of glossy-haired 'clean eating' ladies as you can get, but I think they're onto something with their spiralized vegetables. Don't laugh! The spiralizer is really just a posh grater. It makes great salads and 'noodles'. I particularly like the cool, crunchy spiralized radish in my seared tuna, white radish and sesame salad (page 74); it carries the dressing so beautifully, it's almost addictive.

I hope you'll enjoy the salads in this chapter as much as I've enjoyed devising them. They're mostly speedy to make and all completely delicious to eat. In fact, they've become some of my favourite everyday dishes.

Toasting nuts and seeds

If I feel a salad needs a little extra something, whether it's flavour or crunch, it's often a sprinkling of nuts or seeds I reach for, and roasting or toasting them adds another layer of flavour which can lift even the simplest salad. For seeds, simply toast them in a dry frying pan until they're golden and really fragrant. For nuts, follow the instructions on page 202. It takes just a few minutes and it's certainly worth that bit of extra effort – they're not just delicious, nuts are dopamine boosters too.

Greek salad with nasturtium pesto

Use the freshest and best ingredients you can get your hands on for this stunning salad. Nasturtium leaves are popular in fashionable restaurants, not just because they look great but also because they pack a peppery kick that's very similar to rocket. You can sometimes get them from farmers' markets and veg box schemes, but they are very easy to grow – we can even manage them in the car park at The Hand and Flowers! Alternatively, use fiery, young rocket leaves instead.

Serves: 4

Carb count: 17g per person

2 red peppers, halved, cored and deseeded

2 green peppers, halved, cored and deseeded

2 red onions

2 tomatoes, cored and deseeded

½ cucumber, peeled, halved and deseeded

20 black olives, pitted and sliced

2 tbsp capers

200g best-quality feta cheese, crumbled

1 garlic clove, grated

2 tbsp pine nuts

2 handfuls of nasturtium leaves (about 225g), plus extra to finish

170ml good-quality extra virgin olive oil

1 tbsp red wine vinegar

1 banana shallot, sliced into thin rings

Flaky sea salt and freshly ground black pepper

1 Cut the peppers, red onions, tomatoes and cucumber into 1.5cm dice and place them all in a large bowl. Add the olives and capers and mix together.

2 Using a large pestle and mortar or a food processor, crush 50g of the feta cheese with the garlic and pine nuts to a paste.

3 Gradually work in a couple of handfuls of nasturtium leaves and 140ml olive oil to make a coarse pesto – it should have some texture to it. Season with salt and pepper to taste.

4 Tip the diced salad vegetables into a serving bowl. Dress with the remaining 2 tbsp olive oil and the wine vinegar, and sprinkle with some flaky sea salt.

5 Add the remaining feta to the salad and spoon on the nasturtium pesto. Scatter over the shallot rings, top with some nasturtium leaves and serve.

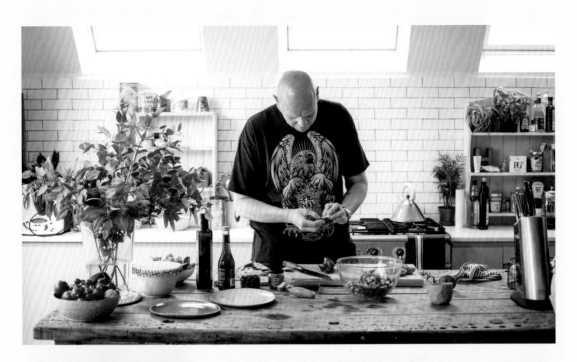

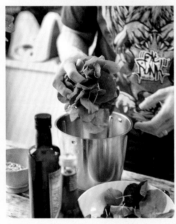

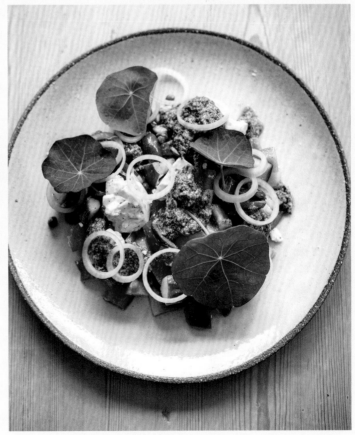

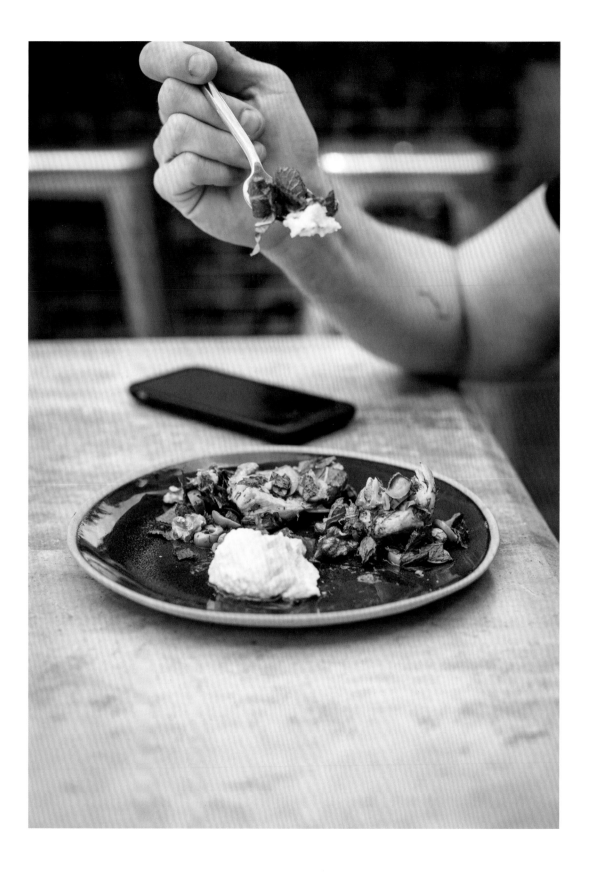

Marinated artichokes with feta and mint

Artichokes, olives and feta cheese: this fantastic salad reminds me of lazy, easy lunches on summer holidays in Greece. I've used whipped feta here. It's simple to make and versatile – add chopped herbs, spices and/or toasted seeds to vary the flavour. Try dolloping it on tomato salads, use it as a dip for crudités or toss it through spiralized courgette noodles.

Serves: 4

Carb count: 16g per person

75g shelled walnuts
300g marinated artichokes in olive oil
100g good-quality green olives, pitted and sliced
2 pickled green chillies, chopped
2 bunches of mint (about 50–60g in total), tough stems removed, leaves roughly chopped
½ bunch of dill (about 10g), chopped
400g best-quality feta cheese
4 tbsp single cream
1 tbsp clear honey
Finely grated zest of 1 lemon

1 To toast the walnuts, either warm them in a frying pan over a medium heat until they are very fragrant and have taken on some colour, or scatter on a baking tray and bake in an oven preheated to 180°C/Fan 160°C/Gas 4 for 8–10 minutes. Be careful not to burn them, but make sure they are well toasted, as it's their texture and flavour that make this salad so fantastic. Set aside to cool.

2 Drain the artichokes, reserving 4–5 tbsp of the oil. Cut the artichokes in half lengthways and place in a large bowl with the olives and pickled chillies. Add the chopped mint and dill and toss to mix.

3 Break the walnuts up with your hands, but not too much – you still want them to give plenty of texture to the finished dish. Add them to the salad and toss to combine then divide between serving plates.

4 In a food processor, blend the feta cheese with the single cream until smooth. Spoon the whipped feta next to the salad.

5 Whisk together the honey, lemon zest and reserved olive oil to make a dressing. Drizzle all over the salad and serve.

Roasted onion salad with fried halloumi

Sometimes the simplest flavours are the best – in my book, you can't beat the classic combination of cheese and onion. Here, they go together to form a great stand-alone salad, but feel free to serve it with roast chicken or pork if you like.

Serves: 4–6

Carb count: 22–15g per person

4 banana shallots, skin on and
     root end intact
Olive oil, for frying
3 medium onions, skin on and
     root end intact
200ml chicken stock
50g butter
2 medium leeks, dark green part
     trimmed away
2 tbsp lemon thyme leaves
2 x 225g packets of halloumi
     cheese, cut into 2cm slices
1 Romaine lettuce, roughly cut
     into pieces
A bunch of spring onions, trimmed
     and cut into 2cm pieces
1 tbsp red wine vinegar
4 tbsp salad cream
A bunch of chives (about 15g),
     finely chopped
Sea salt and freshly ground
     black pepper

1 Preheat the oven to 180°C/Fan 160°C/Gas 4. Cut the shallots in half lengthways, keeping the root end intact.

2 Heat a splash of olive oil in an ovenproof non-stick frying pan over a medium heat. Add the shallots, cut side down, and cook for 8–10 minutes until slightly softened and caramelised. Remove the shallots from the pan and set aside on a plate; keep the frying pan on the heat.

3 Halve the onions through the equator then place, cut side down, in the pan. Cook for about 10 minutes until the cut sides are caramelised. You may need to add more oil. When they have taken on a lovely colour, turn the onions over and add the stock to the pan.

4 Transfer the frying pan to the oven and cook for 15–20 minutes, until the onions have softened and the stock has reduced right down. Remove from the oven and set aside to cool, leaving the oven switched on.

5 In a frying pan, melt the butter along with 100ml water and add some salt and pepper. Cut the leeks in half if they're too long to fit in the pan. Add the leeks to the buttery liquor and simmer gently, turning frequently, until softened. This will take 5–8 minutes. Remove the leeks from the pan, leave to cool then cut into chunks.

6 Next, remove the onions from their skins but keep them whole. Keeping the root end intact, gently pull the shallots apart so they form 'petals'. Place the onions, shallots and leeks on a baking tray. Scatter over the thyme leaves and mix well then warm through in the oven for about 10 minutes.

7 Meanwhile, heat a splash of olive oil in a non-stick frying pan over a medium-high heat and fry the halloumi slices until crisp and golden on both sides, about 2–3 minutes per side. Drain on kitchen paper.

8 Place the lettuce and spring onions in a large bowl. Add the cooked onions, shallots, leeks and halloumi and drizzle with the wine vinegar. Toss to combine, then add the salad cream and chives and toss again. Serve immediately.

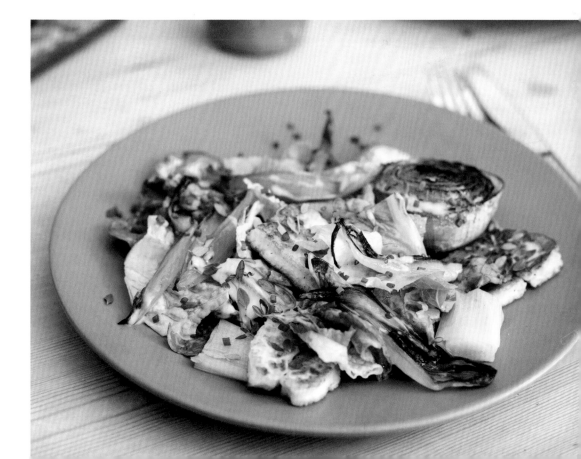

Crispy kale with anchovies and lemon

For me, this version of Chinese crispy 'seaweed' is pretty addictive. I serve it as a side dish, or sometimes I leave out the anchovies and eat it as a snack. Kale's become fashionable for a reason – it's a nutritional powerhouse. It's also full of the good stuff that helps your brain to produce dopamine and is just the thing when you're craving big, strong flavours.

Serves: 4 as a side dish

Carb count: 1g per person

300g kale, tough stalks removed
Vegetable oil, for deep-frying
2 tsp sea salt
1 chicken stock cube
Finely grated zest of 1 lemon
15–20 anchovy fillets in oil,
    drained

1 Tear the kale leaves into largish pieces, rinse well and pat dry with kitchen paper. The kale must be completely dry. (This water-dense vegetable, even when dry, will spit and bubble up dramatically in the pan as you fry it.)

2 Heat the oil in a deep-fryer or other deep, heavy-bottomed pan to 180°C; the pan must be no more than one-third full. Check the temperature with a cook's thermometer.

3 While the oil is heating up, using a pestle and mortar, grind the salt and stock cube together to a fine powder.

4 Place a large tray lined with several layers of kitchen paper next to the deep-fryer or pan.

5 Deep-fry the kale in batches until crisp and translucent, about a minute. Don't overcrowd the pan and step back as you drop the kale in (use tongs), as it will spit ferociously for a few seconds. Once cooked, carefully remove the kale and drain on the kitchen paper, then dust with the stock powder. Repeat the frying and seasoning until all of the kale is cooked.

6 Scatter the lemon zest over the kale then gently transfer to a serving bowl. Interweave the anchovy fillets with the crispy kale and serve straight away.

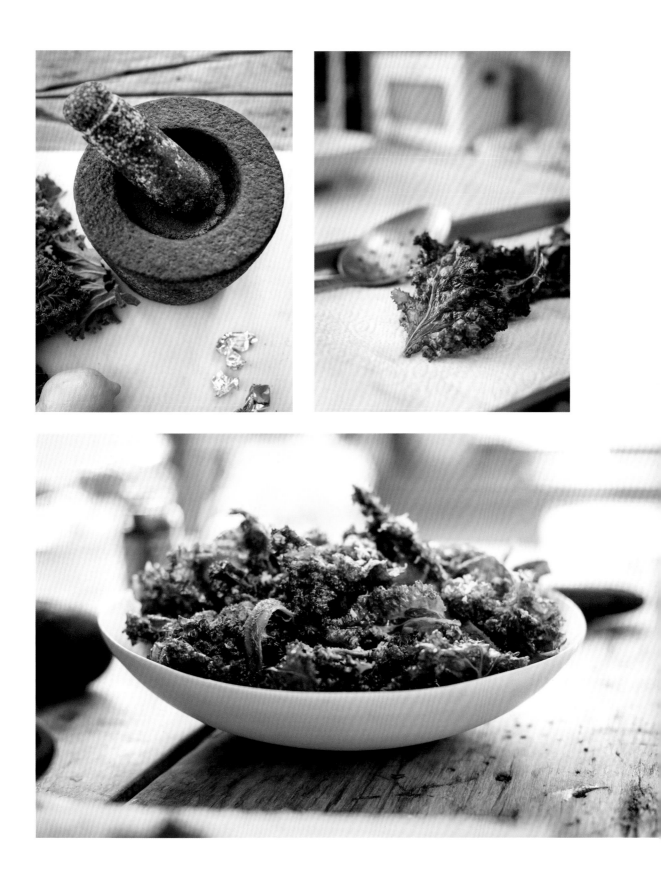

Provençal pickled fish, fennel and orange salad

This is a great summer dish, perfect for a light lunch and outdoor eating. You might not be in the South of France, but the poached fish, fragrant fennel and bittersweet mustard and orange dressing give this recipe a lovely holiday feel.

Serves: 4

Carb count: 16g per person

For the fish:
1 orange
100ml white wine vinegar
1 tbsp demerara sugar
2 star anise
2 cloves
4 gilt-head bream fillets, trimmed, descaled and pin boned (get your fishmonger to do this for you)

For the salad:
2 fennel bulbs
1 tsp flaky sea salt
2 tbsp fennel seeds, lightly toasted in a dry frying pan until fragrant
1 tbsp mustard seeds, lightly toasted in a dry frying pan just until they start to pop
2 oranges
150ml extra virgin olive oil
2 tsp Dijon mustard
2 heads of Little Gem lettuce, finely shredded
A small handful of dill, chopped

1 For the fish, use a sharp vegetable peeler to finely pare the zest off the orange in long strips, being careful not to include the bitter white pith. Halve the orange and squeeze the juice; set this juice aside to use in the salad.

2 Pour 200ml water into a wide, shallow pan or roasting tin and add the wine vinegar, demerara sugar, star anise, cloves and pared orange zest. Bring to a simmer and place the fish fillets in the liquor, then take the pan off the heat. Cover tightly with cling film and put to one side; keep warm.

3 To prepare the salad, using a mandoline, thinly slice the fennel into a bowl. Add the flaky sea salt and massage it into the fennel for 1 minute. Leave to stand for 3–4 minutes to soften a little then pour off any liquid that has accumulated. Add the toasted fennel and mustard seeds. Finely grate over the zest from the oranges.

4 Next, segment both oranges: trim off the top and bottom and stand the fruit on a board. Work your way around the oranges with a small, sharp knife, cutting off the peel, pith and outer membrane. Over a bowl, cut between the membranes to release the segments into the bowl. Squeeze the membranes to extract any remaining juice.

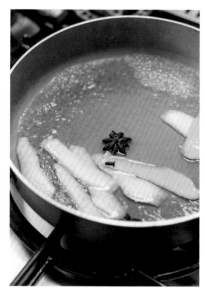

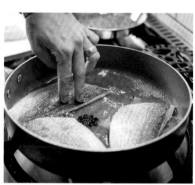

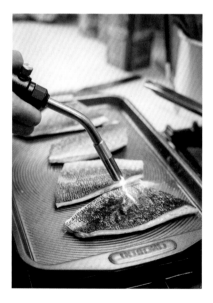

5 Pour all the reserved orange juice into a small pan and let bubble over a medium heat until reduced and thickened to a glaze. Whisk in the olive oil and mustard to make a dressing.

6 Toss the lettuce, dill and orange segments with the fennel.

7 Lift the fish out of the warm poaching liquid and place them, skin side up, on an oven tray. Use a cook's blowtorch to crisp up the skin, or briefly place under a very hot grill.

8 Dress the fennel salad with most of the warm dressing. Divide between serving plates, add a fish fillet to each and drizzle the remaining dressing around.

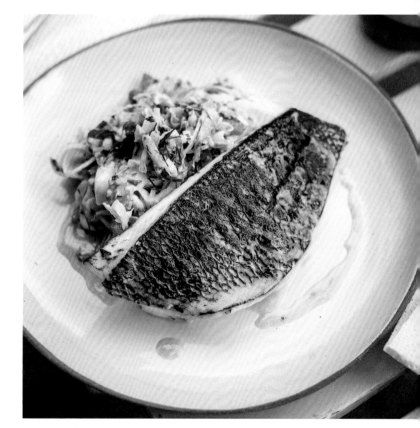

Padrón peppers, anchovy dip and onion crunch

I like to serve this in three separate bowls, so you can dip the scalded peppers into the anchovy dip and then roll them in the onion and pork scratching crumbs before eating. This sort of dish convinces me that chilli heat is addictive.

Serves: 4–6

Carb count: 12–8g per person

For the anchovy dip:
4 tbsp olive oil
4 banana shallots, finely diced
2 garlic cloves, grated
20 anchovy fillets in olive oil, drained
1 tbsp crème fraîche
½ tsp cayenne pepper
40g Parmesan cheese, freshly grated

For the onion crunch:
75g pork scratchings, crushed to a coarse powder
4 tbsp dried onion flakes
2 tsp garlic powder
½ tsp ground cumin

For the peppers:
Olive oil, for frying
400g padrón peppers
Flaky sea salt

1 First, make the anchovy dip. Warm the olive oil in a frying pan over a medium-low heat. Add the shallots and garlic and sweat gently, stirring from time to time, until softened, about 10–15 minutes. Add the anchovies, crème fraîche and cayenne pepper and cook, stirring, for 2–3 minutes until the anchovies start to break down.

2 Remove from the heat and stir in the grated Parmesan. Transfer the mixture to a food processor and blend to a paste. If you're not using it immediately, spoon into a container and keep in the fridge until needed.

3 Preheat the oven to 160°C/Fan 140°C/Gas 3. Mix together the crushed pork scratchings, onion flakes, garlic powder and ground cumin. Scatter on an oven tray and bake until toasted, about 10–12 minutes, stirring once or twice during cooking. Set aside to cool.

4 When you're almost ready to serve, heat a heavy-bottomed cast-iron skillet or non-stick frying pan over a high heat. Drizzle on a little olive oil and then, when it's just smoking hot, add a couple of handfuls of the peppers and cook for 2–3 minutes until blistered and softened. Sprinkle with salt and transfer to a bowl. Repeat with the remaining peppers.

5 Dip the peppers into the anchovy paste then roll in the onion crunch and eat immediately.

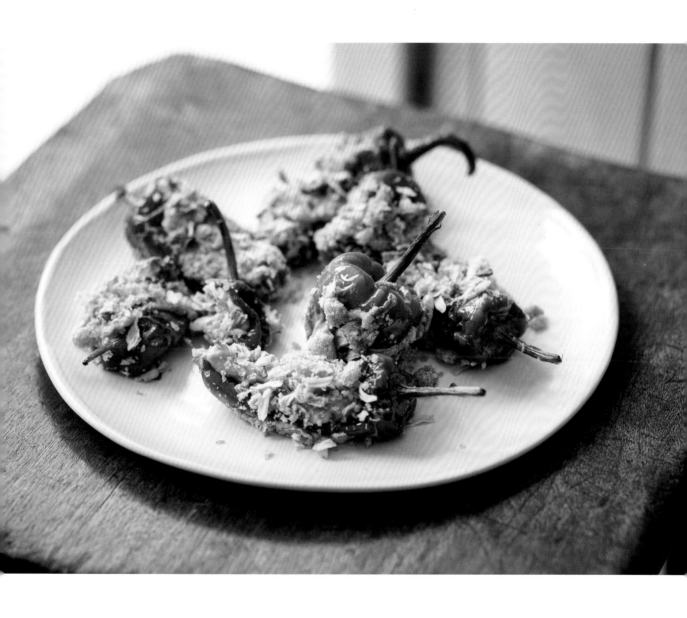

Seared tuna, white radish and sesame salad ⏱

You'll need a spiralizer to turn the white radish into noodles, but once you taste this fiery, cool and crunchy salad you'll realise it's a great investment. You can use salmon or mackerel in place of the tuna if you like.

Serves: 2

Carb count: 14g per person

For the salad:
½ white radish, also called daikon or mooli (about 150g), peeled
Vegetable oil, for frying
2 x 200g pieces of sushi-grade tuna loin
¼ cucumber, thinly sliced
⅓ bunch of coriander (about 10g), chopped, tender stems and all
2 sheets of nori seaweed, cut into 2cm squares
2 tbsp sesame seeds, toasted until golden in a dry frying pan
2 tbsp chopped pickled ginger
Sea salt and freshly ground black pepper

For the dressing:
1 tbsp dark soy sauce
1 tbsp rice wine vinegar
1½ tsp wasabi paste
1 tsp clear honey
2 tbsp olive oil
1 tsp sesame oil

1 Have ready a bowl of heavily iced water. Use a spiralizer to turn the white radish into noodles. Immerse in the iced water for 10–15 minutes until they are crisp and very cold.

2 For the dressing, in a small bowl, whisk together the soy sauce, rice wine vinegar, wasabi and honey, followed by the olive oil and sesame oil. Set aside.

3 Heat a non-stick frying pan over a medium-high heat and then add a splash of oil. Season the tuna with salt and pepper and sear all over – just until the surface is a nice, toasty brown colour; make sure you don't overcook it. Remove from the pan and leave to rest for 2–3 minutes.

4 Drain the noodles and place them on a clean tea towel or on several layers of kitchen paper, to get rid of the excess moisture.

5 Tip the noodles into a large bowl and combine them with the cucumber, coriander, nori squares, sesame seeds and pickled ginger.

6 Toss the salad with the dressing and divide between two plates. Slice the tuna, arrange it next to the salad and serve.

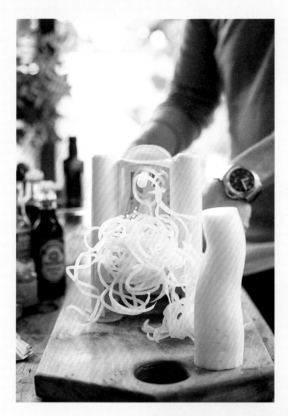

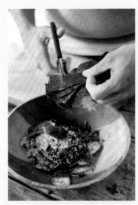

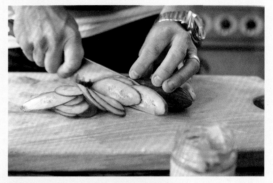

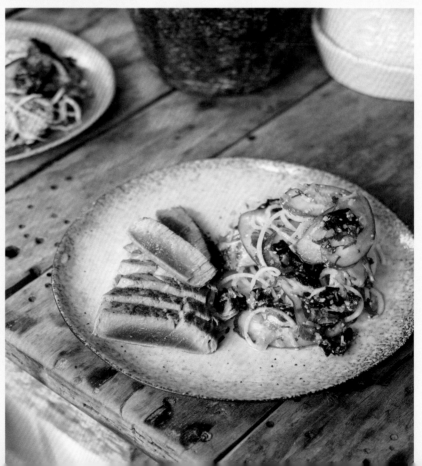

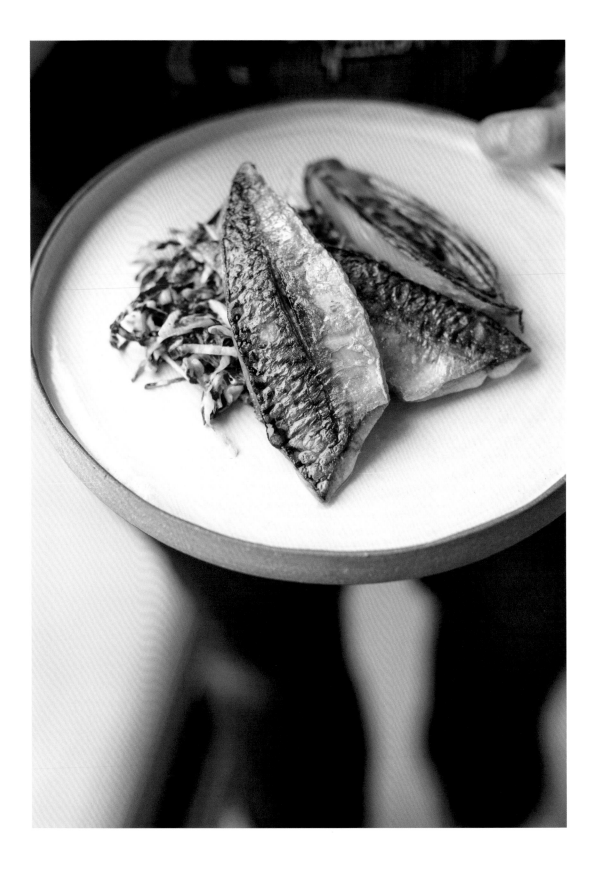

Mackerel, chicory and radicchio Caesar salad ⏱

You can adapt this salad in so many ways. The beautiful, bitter leaves are great with oily fish, but they also work with steak, lamb and chicken. You'll have more dressing than you need for the salad but it will keep in a jar in the fridge for a few days and is great with many veg – try it with roasted cauliflower, or as a dip for crudités or steamed artichoke leaves.

Serves: 2

Carb count: 12g per person

2–3 tbsp olive oil, for cooking
4 mackerel fillets
1 large chicory bulb, halved
	lengthways
A knob of butter
Juice of 1 lemon

For the salad:
1 radicchio, finely shredded
1 tbsp pine nuts, toasted until
	golden in a dry frying pan
1 tbsp chopped tarragon
Finely grated zest of ½ orange

For the Caesar dressing:
1 free-range egg yolk
3 anchovy fillets in oil, drained
1 garlic clove, grated
1½ tsp Dijon mustard
½ tbsp white wine vinegar
150ml fridge-cold vegetable oil
45g Parmesan cheese, freshly
	grated
1 tbsp lemon juice
Cayenne pepper, to taste

1 For the dressing, put the egg yolk, anchovies, garlic, mustard and wine vinegar in a blender or food processor and blitz until smooth. With the motor still running, slowly add the cold oil until the mixture emulsifies. Stir in the grated Parmesan and lemon juice and season with cayenne pepper. Transfer to a container, seal and refrigerate if you're not using it right away.

2 For the salad, put the radicchio, pine nuts, tarragon and orange zest into a large bowl. Add 2–3 tbsp of the dressing and toss to coat.

3 Heat a non-stick frying pan over a medium-high heat and add a generous splash of olive oil. When hot, lay the mackerel fillets in the pan, skin side down, and fry without moving until crisp around the edges, 2–3 minutes. Remove from the pan; the fillets may still be raw on top.

4 Place the chicory in the hot frying pan, cut side down, adding a little more oil if needed. Cook for 2–3 minutes, until it starts to colour. Add the butter then return the fish to the pan, skin side up. Add the lemon juice. Baste the fish and chicory with the lemony, buttery liquor, then remove and drain on kitchen paper.

5 Divide the radicchio, chicory and fish between plates and serve with the remaining dressing.

The Dope: <u>Avocados</u> are creamy
and rich – great in salads and 'wraps'
like this, or whizzed up into dressings
and smoothies.

Chicken, avocado and lettuce wraps

This fast, fresh-tasting recipe makes good use of store-cupboard ingredients. The secret is to get the chicken lovely and crisp on the outside and to eat it as soon as you've wrapped it in the crunchy iceberg lettuce. It makes a great quick lunch.

Serves: 4

Carb count: 11g per person

1 tsp smoked paprika
1 tsp chilli powder
1 tsp salt
4 free-range skinless chicken breasts
2 tbsp vegetable oil
2 avocados
Finely grated zest and juice of 1 lime
2 tbsp Worcestershire sauce
1 tbsp crème fraîche
2 jarred roasted red peppers, chopped
2 pickled green chillies, chopped
2 tbsp chopped coriander, tender stems and all
2 red chillies, sliced, seeds and all (optional)
1 iceberg lettuce, leaves separated from the core and kept whole
Sea salt and freshly ground black pepper

1 In a small bowl, mix together the smoked paprika, chilli powder and salt. Coat the chicken breasts in the seasoning mixture.

2 Heat a non-stick frying pan over a medium heat then add the oil. When hot, place the chicken breasts in the pan and cook, without moving them, for 10–12 minutes, until crisp on the underside. They should be cooked 90 per cent through.

3 Meanwhile, peel, halve, stone and roughly cut up the avocados. Tip them into a bowl and crush with a fork. Add the lime zest and juice, Worcestershire sauce and crème fraîche. Mix thoroughly and season with salt and pepper.

4 In another bowl, mix the red peppers with the pickled green chillies and coriander, adding the red chillies too, if you fancy the extra heat.

5 Turn the chicken breasts over in the pan and cook for a further 3–4 minutes until cooked through. Transfer to a board and leave to rest for 5 minutes, then cut into 1cm pieces and combine with the red pepper mixture.

6 Spread some avocado onto a lettuce leaf, add some of the chicken mix, then roll the lettuce up like a cigar to make a wrap. Repeat with the remaining ingredients. Eat immediately. Supply paper napkins – this is messy food!

Steak, red onion and tomato salad

I love beef and tomatoes together. The sweet acidity of the tomatoes combined with the salty, meaty crust on the steak works brilliantly in this salad. It's ideal if you want to get something really appetising on the table quickly. Bavette, sometimes called skirt steak, has a fantastic flavour and is great value for money but it can be tough if you overcook it, so make sure you keep it nice and pink. Of course, you can swap the bavette for sirloin or rib eye if you prefer.

Serves: 2

Carb count: 14g per person

4 plum tomatoes, thinly sliced
1 small red onion, halved and
    thinly sliced
½ tsp cracked black pepper
Vegetable oil, for cooking
2 bavette steaks (250g each)
20g butter
Juice of ½ lemon
1 ball of mozzarella (about 125g),
    drained and diced
½ bunch of basil (about 15g),
    large stems discarded
2 tbsp roughly chopped sun-dried
    tomatoes
1 red chilli, thinly sliced, seeds
    and all
1 tbsp best-quality balsamic
    vinegar
¾ tbsp extra virgin olive oil
Flaky sea salt
25g Parmesan cheese, to finish

1 Arrange the sliced tomatoes on a large serving plate. Scatter over the red onion, sprinkle with half of the cracked black pepper and season with salt to taste.

2 Heat a splash of oil in a frying pan over a medium-high heat. Season the steaks with salt and the remaining cracked pepper and place them in the hot pan. Add the butter and let it brown and colour the steaks well. This will take 4–5 minutes. Flip the steaks over, add the lemon juice and cook, basting the meat with the lemony butter, for 1–2 minutes.

3 Lift the steaks out of the frying pan onto a warm plate and leave to rest in a warm place for 10 minutes.

4 Drain off any liquid from the tomato plate. Scatter the mozzarella, basil leaves, sun-dried tomatoes and chilli over the tomatoes.

5 Slice the beef against the grain and arrange it over the tomato salad. Pour over any juices that have accumulated on the steak plate too.

6 Mix the balsamic vinegar and olive oil together and drizzle all over the salad. Grate over the Parmesan just before serving.

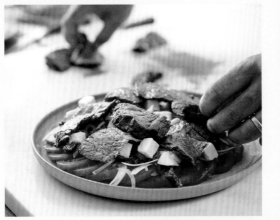

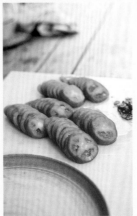

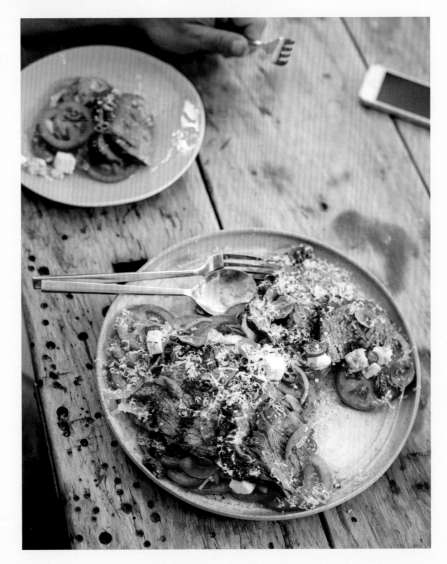

Spinach, sesame and pork scratchings salad

This is a great little lunch dish. Crunchy, spiced pork scratchings are deliciously tempered by the richness of salty Roquefort, wilted leaves and silky duck egg yolk. The scratchings make a brilliant snack so you might want to make a double batch. I like them quite hot, but if you'd prefer them a bit milder, use less cayenne and chilli powder. You won't need all of the dressing but it makes an excellent dip for crudités so keep the rest in a jar in the fridge, for up to 4 days.

Serves: 4
Carb count: 1g per person

For the hot pork scratchings:
1 tsp cayenne pepper
1 tsp curry powder
1 tsp chilli powder
½ tsp ground cumin
150g pork scratchings

For the dressing:
1 tbsp tahini
1 free-range egg yolk
1 tbsp brown malt vinegar
120ml olive oil
30ml sesame oil
3 tbsp sesame seeds, lightly toasted in a dry frying pan until just golden

For the salad:
20g butter
200g baby spinach
2 tbsp vegetable oil
4 free-range duck eggs
100g rocket leaves
150g Roquefort cheese, crumbled

1 Preheat the oven to 180°C/Fan 160°C/Gas 4. For the hot pork scratchings, mix the ground spices with 2–3 tbsp water to make a paste. Add the pork scratchings and stir to coat evenly. Transfer to an oven tray and roast in the oven for 5–10 minutes. Drain and cool on kitchen paper.

2 For the dressing, beat together the tahini, egg yolk and vinegar in a bowl until well combined. Slowly whisk in the olive oil, then the sesame oil to emulsify. Add a little hot water to thin the dressing to the consistency of double cream. Stir in the sesame seeds.

3 Warm the butter in a large frying pan over a medium-low heat. When it has melted and stops foaming, add the spinach and cook gently just until wilted.

The Dope: Spinach is one of the most versatile leaves there is. You can consume handfuls of it raw in salads, or transform it into a silky, luxurious purée when cooked.

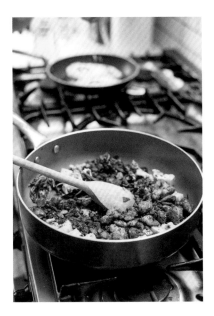

4 Meanwhile, heat the oil in another large frying pan. When it's hot, fry the duck eggs over a high heat until the whites are cooked and a bit crispy around the edges. Remove the eggs from the pan and place on a warmed plate.

5 Mix the rocket with the wilted spinach and dress with just enough sesame dressing to coat.

6 Toss half the spicy pork scratchings through the dressed leaves and gently fold in the soft, crumbly Roquefort.

7 Divide the salad between four plates, put a fried egg on top of each serving and scatter over the rest of the pork scratchings to serve.

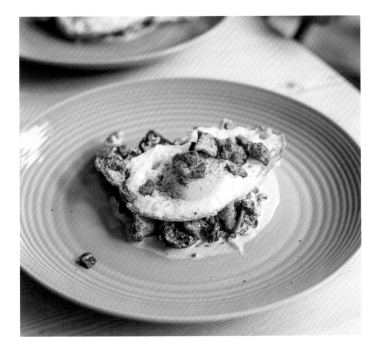

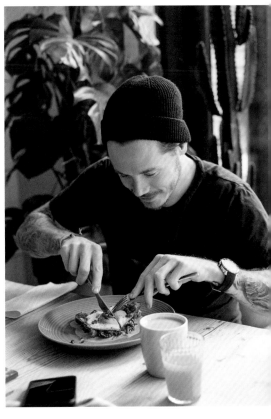

Pickled pork with turnip and seaweed salad

There are all kinds of flavours and textures going on in this unusual and highly delicious salad. It takes a little planning ahead – ideally, you should let the pork sit in the pickling liquid overnight, or at least for 3 or 4 hours – but none of it is very complicated. Salty seaweed, slightly bitter turnips and sweet-sour pickled pork is a cracking combination. Give it a go!

Serves: 4
Carb count: 13g per person

For the pickled pork belly:
750g piece of boned pork belly
1½ tsp salt, plus extra for rubbing
    into the pork skin
200ml white wine vinegar
2 celery sticks, trimmed and halved
6 garlic cloves, lightly crushed
3 bay leaves
1 tbsp demerara sugar

For the turnip and seaweed salad:
60g packet of dried wakame
    seaweed
4 large turnips (about 150–200g
    each)
3 tbsp extra virgin olive oil
A bunch of spring onions, trimmed
    and sliced
A bunch of coriander (about 30g),
    any tough stalks removed,
    coarsely chopped
2 tbsp yellow mustard seeds,
    lightly toasted in a dry frying
    pan until starting to pop
2 tbsp sesame seeds, lightly
    toasted in a dry frying pan
    until just golden
2 tbsp Sriracha sauce
1 tbsp white wine vinegar
1 tbsp dark soy sauce
1 tbsp sesame oil
1 tsp freshly grated ginger

1 Preheat the oven to 180°C/Fan 160°C/Gas 4. Remove the skin from the pork belly. Score the skin, if the butcher hasn't already done it for you, then rub it with a little salt. Lay it on a rack in a roasting tin, with a second rack on top to prevent the pork skin from curling. Bake until it puffs up into crunchy crackling, removing the top rack after 30 minutes. It should take 45 minutes–1 hour. Remove and leave to cool. Turn the oven down to 150°C/Fan 130°C/Gas 2.

2 Pour the wine vinegar and 400ml water into a casserole and add the celery, garlic, bay leaves, demerara sugar and 1½ tsp salt. Bring to a simmer. Place the pork belly in the pan and put the lid on. Turn the heat down to a very low simmer and then transfer the casserole to the oven. Cook for 2 hours.

3 Remove the casserole from the oven but don't lift the lid. Leave the pork belly to cool in the liquor for at least 3–4 hours, but preferably overnight. If you're leaving it overnight, once the pan is completely cold, place it in the fridge. The next day take it out of the fridge a couple of hours before you want to serve it.

4 For the salad, soak the dried seaweed in a bowl of cold water for 20 minutes to soften.

⑤ Meanwhile, peel the turnips and use a mandoline to slice them as thinly as possible.

⑥ Drain the seaweed, place in a saucepan and warm gently. Add the olive oil, spring onions, coriander, mustard and sesame seeds, then stir in the Sriracha sauce, wine vinegar, soy, sesame oil and ginger. Add the turnips, toss well and take off the heat.

⑦ Remove the pork from its liquor and cut into slices, about 5mm thick; it should be served at room temperature. Break up the crackling. Arrange the pork and salad on serving plates, scatter over the crackling and serve.

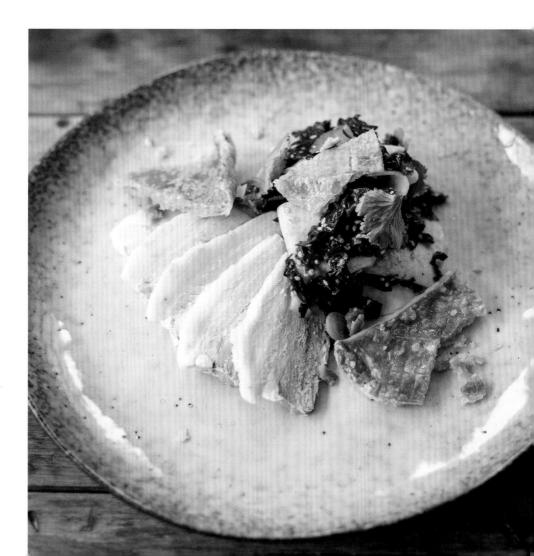

Ham with cucumber and dill pickle salad

This is my ultimate quick lunch or supper dish: a wonderful slab of salty ham spiked with heat from mustard seeds and black pepper, with a nice, tangy cucumber and dill pickle salad on the side. It ticks every box! To make it even more substantial, I sometimes top it with a fried egg.

Serves: 2

Carb count: 18g per person

100ml dill pickle liquor, strained from the pickle jar
50g butter
2 tbsp yellow mustard seeds
1 tbsp cracked black pepper
2 thick slices of good butcher's ham (200–250g each)
4 large dill pickles, diced
2 banana shallots, finely diced
¼ cucumber, deseeded and diced
2 pickled green chillies, chopped
½ bunch of dill (about 10g), chopped

1 Pour 100ml water into a large frying pan, add the pickle liquor and butter and bring to the boil. Add the mustard seeds and cracked black pepper then place the slices of ham in the pan and turn the heat down to low. Gently warm the ham through and let the liquid and butter emulsify.

2 While the ham is warming, in a bowl, mix together the dill pickles, shallots, cucumber, chillies and chopped dill.

3 Remove the ham from the pan, making sure each slice has a good coating of mustard seeds and pepper. Serve on warmed plates with the cucumber and dill pickle salad alongside. The ham is also delicious cold.

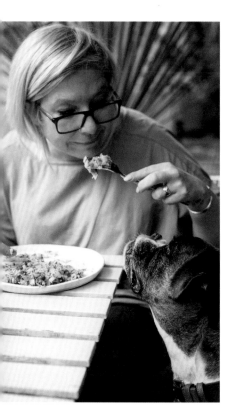
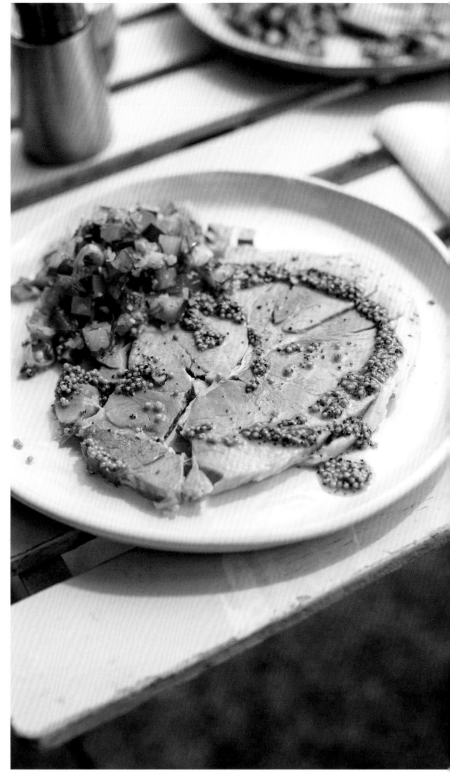

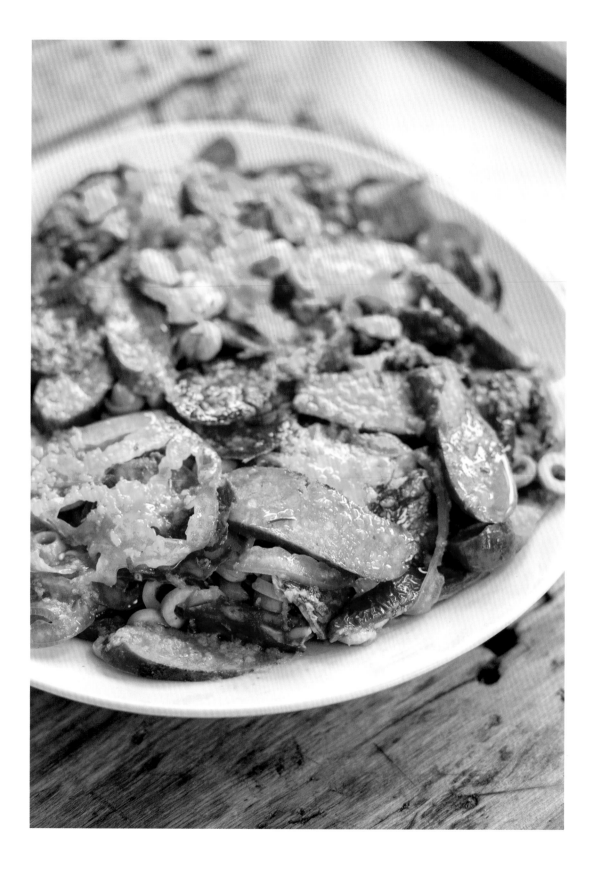

Tomato, chorizo and almond salad

This is a great big substantial plate of warm and spicy 'red' flavours. The tomatoes, chorizo and saffron give it a sunshine feel. As it is very simple, the tomatoes need to be ripe and flavourful, and the olive oil, olives and almonds should be the finest you can lay your hands on. Tomatoes always taste best at room temperature; even storing them in the fridge spoils their flavour and texture.

Serves: 6

Carb count: 13g per person

2 large beefsteak tomatoes
6 plum tomatoes
A splash of dry sherry (about 40ml)
A large pinch of saffron strands
100ml extra virgin olive oil
150g sun-dried tomatoes in oil
    (drained weight, oil reserved),
    halved
4 garlic cloves, grated
200g roasted salted almonds
150g green olives, ideally
    Manzanillo, pitted and sliced
A bunch of sage (about 15g), thick
    stems removed, leaves roughly
    chopped
200g picante dry-cured chorizo,
    thinly sliced
250g whole chorizo sausages
    (for cooking)
Flaky sea salt

1 Slice all the fresh tomatoes very thinly and layer them on a large serving platter. Sprinkle with flaky sea salt and set aside.

2 In a small saucepan, gently warm the sherry with the saffron until the strands release their flavour and colour. Add the olive oil and the oil from the sun-dried tomatoes, and gently heat through for 3–5 minutes. Add the garlic, remove from the heat and leave to cool.

3 Gently mix the roasted almonds, sun-dried tomatoes, olives and chopped sage with the fresh tomatoes. Fold through the cured, sliced chorizo.

4 Warm a non-stick frying pan over a medium heat, add the raw chorizo sausages and cook, turning as necessary, until cooked through. Remove from the pan and slice on an angle then mix into the tomatoes while still warm. Drizzle over the saffron-infused oil and serve.

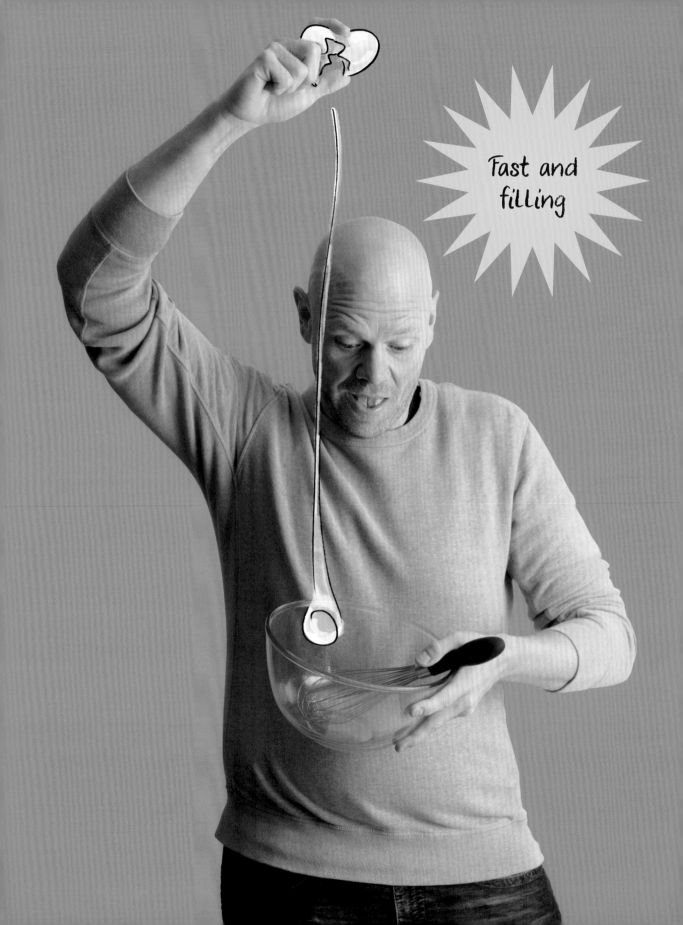

Fast and filling

OMELETTES
&
PANCAKES

F YOU HAVE A BOX OF EGGS and a few odds and ends in the fridge, you're never more than 10 minutes away from a great dinner. Versatile and inexpensive, eggs are high in protein and keep you feeling full and satisfied. They're also a valuable source of vitamins and minerals, and high in the amino acids which help stimulate dopamine production.

For their mood-boosting properties and huge versatility, free-range eggs have become a massive staple of my diet over the past couple of years. Eggs hold flavours, seasonings, spices and herbs brilliantly. Their character is even altered subtly depending on whether you cook them in butter or oil.

When I really got stuck into my new eating regime, I started to think about eggs in the same way as I used to think about pasta. You know when you stand in front of the fridge and think, 'I've got that little bit of ham, a piece of Roquefort, and some broccoli left over from last night's dinner, I can make a tasty pasta dish with what I've got here.' You can use eggs in exactly the same way. They will carry pretty much all of the same flavours and textures to give you a great meal with very little effort.

A fried or poached egg can transform a simple salad or soup into a wholesome meal, and in the form of omelettes, eggs are a sustaining dinner in their own right. I'll admit I get pretty excited about omelettes – they offer such variety. Whether you go for a rich and elegant hot-smoked salmon and chive omelette (page 107) or the earthy chicken forestière omelette (page 115), there's something to suit whatever you're in the mood for.

And then, as an extension of that, there are some wonderful pizza omelettes (on pages 108, 121 and 122). These are so versatile. You can vary the topping ingredients according to what you've got in the fridge and whatever your favourite pizza toppings are. Hold back on the pineapple though – not just because I'm not sure how good egg and pineapple might be – this fruit is high in sugar.

One of the great things about omelettes – whether they're fine and rolled, like the tamagoyaki omelette (page 100), or more substantial one-pan affairs, such as the sausage, sage and onion omelette (page 116) – is that they really do work hot or cold, which makes them very good for packed lunches, either with a salad or on their own. In fact, many other cultures have a tradition of cold omelettes: Spain has its tortilla, Italy its frittata. I think it's about time we laid claim to one of our own, especially as omelettes often taste even more delicious the next day.

What to have for breakfast

When you ditch the habit of tucking into a bowl of cereal or a couple of slices of toast, it can be a challenge to come up with easy, quick, low-carb alternatives. Here are some of the things that work for me:

* Plain wholemilk yoghurt, sometimes with fruit.
* An omelette, either hot or cold – my boil-in-the-bag cheese omelette (page 104) is an easy option.
* A full, cooked breakfast if I've got the time.
* Cold sausages and some good, hot mustard. If I'm cooking sausages for dinner, I do a few extra to have for breakfast the next morning.
* A Turkish-style breakfast of salami, cheese, olives – add a boiled egg if you like.
* Some slices of tyrosine-rich avocado with smoked salmon and a squeeze of lemon.
* Flaxseed biscuits (page 254), cheese and some cherry tomatoes.

Chive pancakes with asparagus

When in season, English asparagus is unrivalled and I'm constantly trying to find new ways to use it. This makes a very quick, tasty lunch dish or light supper. Serve it just as it is, or add ham or crispy bacon for a more substantial meal.

Serves: 2

Carb count: 8g per person

For the pancakes:
5 large free-range eggs
150g cream cheese
2 tbsp chopped chives
Vegetable oil, for cooking
Sea salt and freshly ground
    black pepper

For the filling:
10 asparagus spears
75g butter

For the dressing:
2 free-range eggs, hard-boiled,
    peeled and grated
3 tbsp capers
1 tbsp Dijon mustard
1 tbsp chopped parsley
1 tbsp white wine vinegar
150ml good-quality extra virgin
    olive oil

1. To prepare the asparagus for the filling, cut off the woody ends and peel the lower part of the spears with a sharp vegetable peeler.

2. For the pancakes, whisk together the eggs, cream cheese and chopped chives and season well with salt and pepper.

3. Heat a little oil in a non-stick frying pan over a medium heat. Spoon a quarter of the egg mix into the pan and fry until browned and crispy underneath, then turn and cook the other side. Remove and drain on kitchen paper; keep warm. Repeat with the rest of the mix to make 4 pancakes.

4. Bring the butter and 150ml water to the boil in a frying pan. Season with salt and pepper and then add the asparagus. Simmer gently, moving the spears around now and then, until tender when pierced with a small, sharp knife, about 3–4 minutes.

5. Meanwhile, make the dressing. Mix together the grated boiled eggs, capers, Dijon mustard, parsley and wine vinegar. Stir in the olive oil.

6. Serve a couple of pancakes per person, with the asparagus alongside and the dressing spooned over the top.

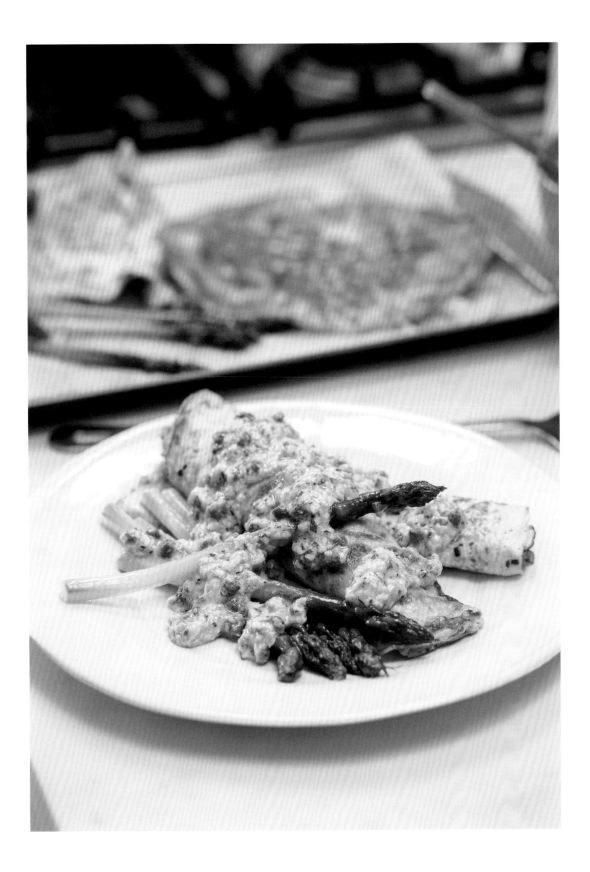

Twice-cooked four-cheese omelette

Make this omelette the day before if possible, so it has lots of time to set and firm up. When you re-fry it the next day, it will become deliciously crispy. The savoury, cheesy taste and crunchy texture makes it one of the best late-night snacks ever.

Serves: 2

Carb count: 14g per person

6 large free-range eggs
1½ tsp English mustard
1 ball of mozzarella (about 125g), drained and torn into small pieces
100g mature Cheddar cheese, grated
100g Stinking Bishop cheese, Époisses or other strong, washed-rind cow's milk cheese, cut into small pieces
3 tbsp ready-made onion marmalade
1 tbsp olive oil
25g butter
100g Parmesan cheese, freshly grated
Vegetable oil, for cooking
A bunch of chives (about 15g), chopped
Sea salt and freshly ground black pepper

① Preheat the oven to 200°C/Fan 180°C/Gas 6. In a bowl, whisk together the eggs, mustard and some salt and pepper. Fold through the mozzarella, Cheddar and Stinking Bishop or Époisses, then stir in the onion marmalade.

② Warm a 24cm non-stick ovenproof frying pan over a medium heat and add the olive oil followed by the butter. When the butter stops foaming, pour in the egg and cheese mixture. Stir around until it starts to thicken, then place the pan in the oven for 12–15 minutes, until the eggs have set completely. Remove from the oven and leave to cool in the pan.

③ After about an hour, carefully remove the omelette from the pan and place on a plate. When it is completely cold, cover with cling film and place in the fridge to set further and chill for a few hours, ideally overnight.

④ Scatter the grated Parmesan on a plate. Cut the omelette into big wedges and press into the cheese to ensure a good covering.

⑤ Heat a non-stick frying pan over a medium heat and add a little oil. Fry the omelette wedges until browned, crispy and thoroughly warmed through. You'll probably need to do this in batches.

⑥ Serve the omelette sprinkled with chives, with a crisp salad on the side if you fancy.

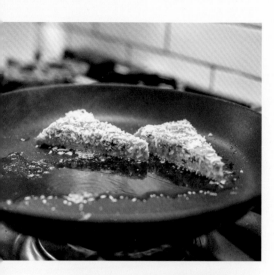

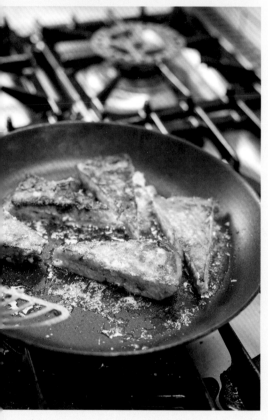

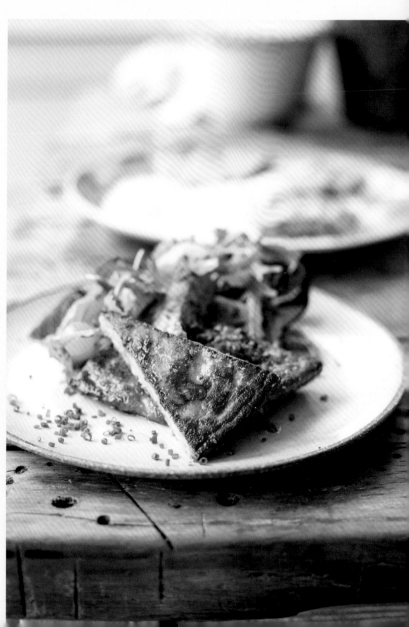

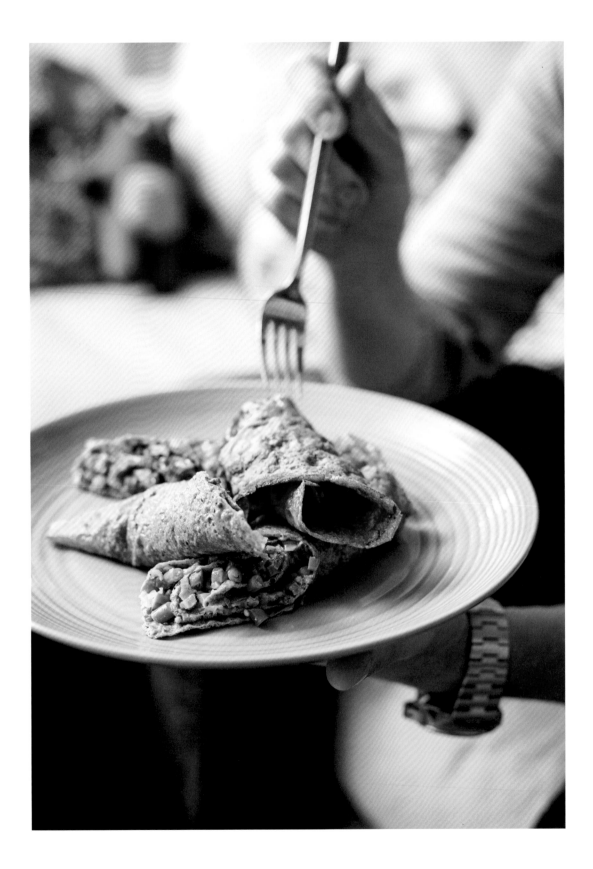

Spicy Indian egg rolls

These rolled-up vegetarian pancakes work well as a carb-alternative side dish with a curry – for those times when you're missing rice or naan bread – but they're equally tasty on their own. They're even good cold for a picnic or packed lunch.

Serves: 2

Carb count: 14g per person

2 tbsp yellow mustard seeds
1 tsp cumin seeds
1 tsp chilli powder
1 tsp cracked black pepper
1 tsp sea salt
½ tsp ground turmeric
½ tsp ground coriander
Vegetable oil, for cooking
4 large free-range eggs
50g butter
1 onion, diced
1 garlic clove, grated
3cm knob of fresh ginger, peeled
    and grated
1 tsp curry powder
200g French beans, chopped
    quite small
10 okra, sliced
2 tbsp chopped coriander leaves

1 In a small bowl, mix the mustard seeds, cumin seeds, chilli powder, cracked pepper, salt, turmeric and ground coriander together. Warm a splash of oil in a frying pan over a medium heat. Add the mixed spices and fry, stirring, for 2–3 minutes until toasted. Take off the heat, add 75ml water and mix to a paste. Let cool.

2 In a bowl, whisk the eggs until evenly blended then add the cooled spice paste and mix until well combined.

3 Warm a 24cm non-stick frying pan over a medium heat, drizzle in a little oil, then ladle in a quarter of the egg mixture, just enough to cover the bottom of the pan. Once set, flip over and cook the other side. Remove and drain on kitchen paper. Repeat with the rest of the egg mixture to make 4 pancakes. Set aside.

4 Melt the butter in a pan over a medium-low heat. When it has stopped foaming, add the onion, garlic and ginger. Sweat gently, stirring occasionally, for 10–15 minutes until soft. Stir in the curry powder then add the French beans and okra and cook, stirring often, for 2–3 minutes. Remove from the heat, stir in the coriander and divide into 4 portions.

5 Spread some of the vegetable mixture on each pancake and roll up. Serve straight away, or reheat later in an oven preheated to 200°C/Fan 180°C/Gas 6 until hot, about 6–8 minutes.

99

Tamagoyaki omelette with pickled radish

I'm not going to lie, Japanese tamagoyaki omelettes take a little practice, but once you get the hang of them, they're great fun to make. It's definitely worth buying a proper, rectangular tamagoyaki pan – they're not expensive. And, if you're unsure about the technique, you'll find tamagoyaki demonstrations on YouTube. With the pickled white radish, this omelette tastes great hot or cold – either on its own or with some sashimi. It makes a good packed lunch with a salad, too.

Serves: 2

Carb count: 18g per person

For the omelette:
4 large free-range eggs, lightly beaten
3 tbsp ready-made dashi stock
1 tbsp mirin (Japanese rice wine)
1 tbsp dark soy sauce
1 tsp erythritol (sugar replacement)
Vegetable oil, for cooking
2 nori sheets, cut in half lengthways

For the pickled radish:
½ white radish, also called daikon or mooli (about 150g), peeled
1 tbsp dark soy sauce
1 tbsp mirin (Japanese rice wine)
1 tbsp sesame oil
1 tbsp vegetable oil
2 tsp grated garlic
2 tsp wasabi paste

To serve (optional):
Very fresh ready-prepared sashimi

1 Pour the beaten eggs into a jug and add the dashi, mirin, soy sauce and erythritol. Mix to combine.

2 Warm the tamagoyaki pan over a low heat and rub the inside with a wad of kitchen paper soaked in vegetable oil.

3 Pour in enough egg mixture just to cover the bottom of the pan. When it's set, lay one of the nori halves on top. Leave to soften for a few seconds, then roll the omelette up towards the handle edge of the pan.

4 Pour a second layer of egg mix into the pan, lifting the rolled omelette slightly to let the egg flow underneath. Cook until it's set then roll up the set egg again, starting with the previously cooked bit of omelette, and rolling towards the opposite edge, away from the pan's handle.

5 Rub the pan with oil again then pour in more egg, lifting up the roll so some egg can flow underneath. Cook until set then add another piece of nori. Leave for a few seconds, then once again roll the whole omelette up like a Swiss roll, towards the handle side of the pan. Keep going until all of the egg mixture and nori is used and the eggs are cooked through.

6 Remove the rolled egg and seaweed 'cigar' from the pan, wrap it in a clean tea towel and roll very tightly. This is the way you get the omelette to take on its nice, tight cylinder shape. You could use a bamboo sushi mat for this instead of the tea towel, if you have one. Leave to rest for 5 minutes.

7 While the omelette is resting, thinly slice or grate the radish. Place in a bowl with the rest of the pickle ingredients and stir to combine.

8 Unwrap the omelette and cut into thick slices. Serve with the pickled white radish, and some sashimi alongside if you fancy.

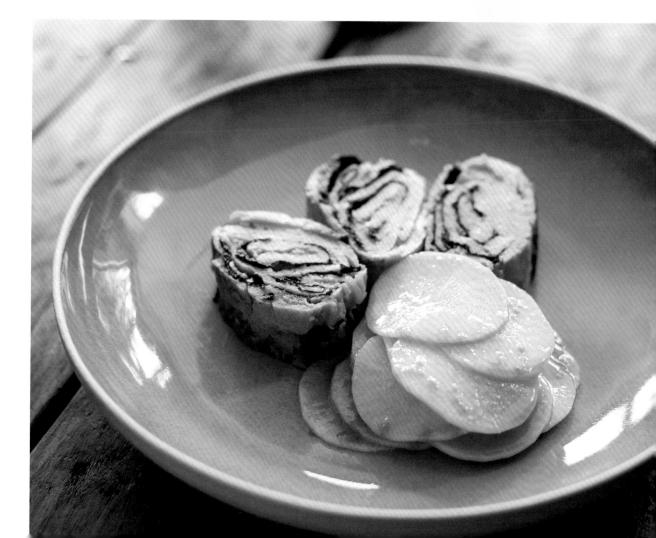

Roasted cauliflower omelette with apple salad 🥫

This recipe transforms simple, everyday ingredients into something very special. The pan-roasted cauliflower and toasted caraway seeds give the rich, cheesy omelette a lovely nutty flavour and the lively, crunchy apple side salad balances the dish perfectly.

Serves: 2–4

Carb count: 24–12g per person

Vegetable oil, for cooking
1 small cauliflower (about 500g), separated into florets and halved lengthways
25g butter
6 large free-range eggs
1 tsp curry powder
½ tsp chilli powder
1 tbsp caraway seeds, lightly toasted in a dry frying pan until just fragrant
100g mature Cheddar cheese, grated
100g Gruyère cheese, grated
Sea salt and freshly ground black pepper

For the apple salad:
1 Granny Smith apple
150g lamb's lettuce
50g rocket leaves
1 tbsp red wine vinegar
3 tbsp extra virgin olive oil

1 Preheat the oven to 180°C/Fan 160°C/Gas 4. Warm a splash of oil in a 24cm non-stick ovenproof frying pan over a medium heat. Add the cauliflower florets, flat side down, and cook until the underside browns and the florets begin to soften. Flip them over, add the butter and cook for a further 3–4 minutes until cooked through. Remove from the heat and flip the cauliflower back onto its flat side.

2 In a bowl, whisk the eggs together with the curry powder, chilli powder and some salt and pepper.

3 Add the caraway seeds to the pan with the cauliflower florets and scatter over the grated cheeses. Place the pan back on a medium heat and then pour in the egg mixture. When it starts to set on the bottom, transfer the pan to the oven and bake for 15–20 minutes.

4 Meanwhile, for the salad, core the apple and slice it into slim batons. Mix together with the lamb's lettuce and rocket.

5 Remove the pan from the oven and leave the omelette to rest for 3–4 minutes.

6 Gently tip the omelette onto a warmed plate. Dress the salad with the wine vinegar and extra virgin olive oil, spoon on top of the omelette and serve immediately.

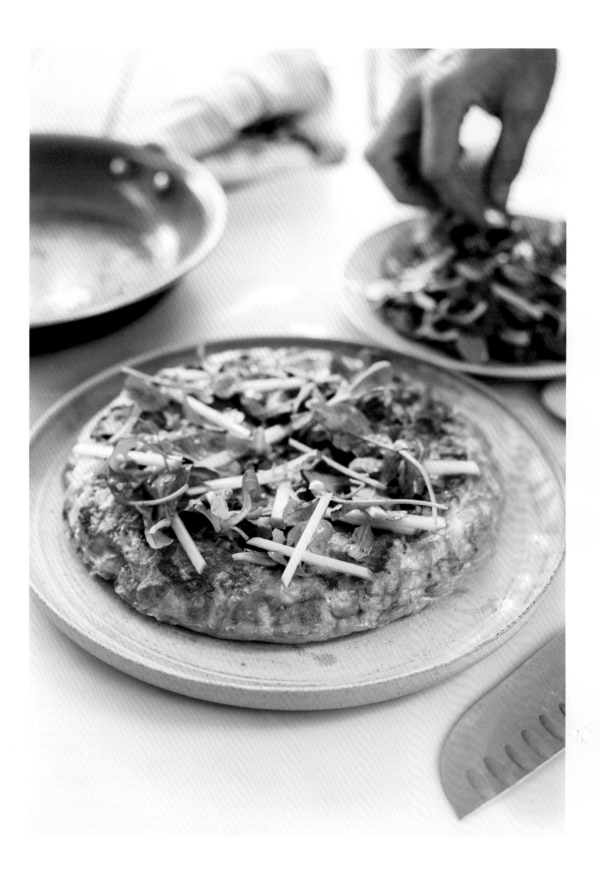

Boil-in-the-bag cheese omelette

I came across this slightly crazy method of cooking eggs while I was filming for the BBC *Food & Drink* programme. The idea was to cook an omelette in a boiling kettle and I was pretty sceptical at first but the result was impressive – an omelette with the perfect soft texture. This is a simple cheese version, but feel free to add herbs, spices, bits of ham and any other layers of flavour that appeal to you.

Serves: 2

Carb count: 1g per person

150g mature Cheddar cheese, grated
4–6 large free-range eggs
50ml double cream
Sea salt and freshly ground black pepper

1. Open two sealable plastic sandwich bags and divide the cheese between the bags.

2. In a bowl, whisk the eggs and cream together and season well with salt and pepper.

3. Carefully pour half of the egg mixture into each of the sandwich bags and seal tightly.

4. Bring a large pan of water to the boil and then turn the heat down so it's just simmering. Add the sealed bags and cook for 8–10 minutes, until the egg mixture is set.

5. Use scissors to cut open the bags, and slide out the cooked omelettes onto plates. Serve at once – they go very well with a full English!

The Dope: Inexpensive, versatile and rich in health-boosting omega-3 fatty acids, eggs have become one of my greatest allies in my new eating programme. They take on almost any seasoning beautifully and make a great, protein-rich meal.

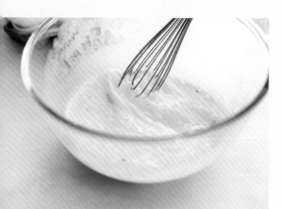

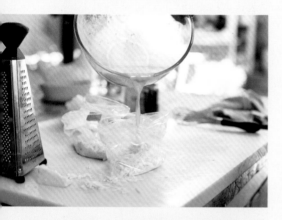

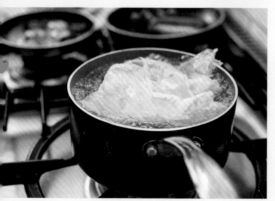

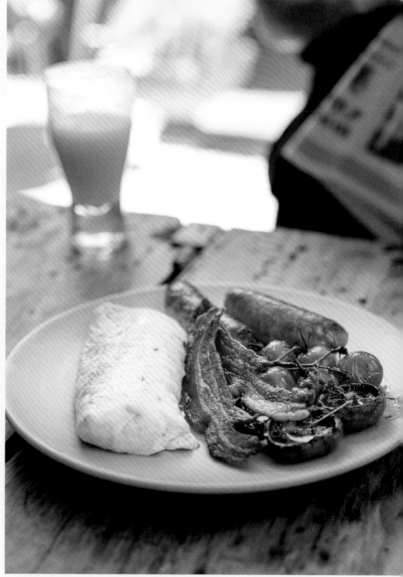

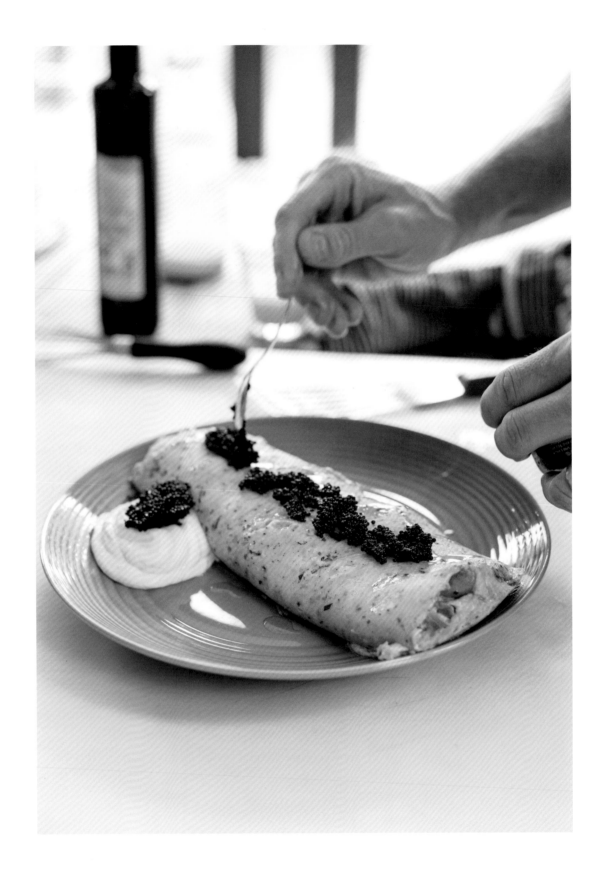

Hot-smoked salmon and chive omelette

The classic combination of smoked salmon and caviar is typically served on carb-heavy blinis, but my omelette version is just as delicious and luxurious. I use flaked, hot-smoked salmon rather than the usual thin slices of smoked salmon, and Avruga caviar – an excellent, less expensive option made from herring roe. Use good-quality French crème fraîche if you can – it makes a big difference here.

Serves: 2

Carb count: 9g per person

6 large free-range eggs
A bunch of chives (about 25g),
    finely chopped
25g butter
200g hot-smoked salmon
2 banana shallots, finely diced
1 ball of mozzarella (about 125g),
    drained and diced
Sea salt and freshly ground
    black pepper

To serve:
4 tbsp good-quality crème fraîche
Finely grated zest of ½ lemon
55g jar Avruga caviar
A drizzle of good-quality extra
    virgin olive oil

1. Preheat the oven to 180°C/Fan 160°C/Gas 4. Whisk the eggs and chives together in a bowl and season with salt and pepper.

2. Melt the butter in a non-stick frying pan over a low heat – don't let it take on any colour. Pour in the beaten egg mixture and cook slowly, moving it around all the time until it starts to thicken and set. Remove the pan from the heat.

3. Flake the hot smoked salmon on top of the omelette, trying not to break it up too much. Scatter on the diced shallots and mozzarella.

4. Roll the omelette up like a cigar and place it in a roasting tin in the oven for 4–5 minutes, just to warm the salmon through and help the mozzarella to melt.

5. Meanwhile, in a bowl, whisk together the crème fraîche and lemon zest until thick.

6. Remove the omelette from the oven and carefully lift it onto a plate. Dollop the lemony crème fraîche alongside, spoon the caviar on top and finish with a trickle of olive oil. Cut the omelette in half and serve some lightly dressed frisée on the side if you like.

Omelette niçoise

This is a big, bold open-faced omelette, inspired by the Provençal flavours of a classic *salade niçoise*. Feel free to swap the tinned tuna for fresh, sushi-grade tuna loin – cooked very pink and thinly sliced.

Serves: 2
Carb count: 6g per person

For the omelette:
50g cherry tomatoes, halved
40g French beans, cooked and
    finely chopped
1 banana shallot, finely diced
¼ small cucumber, deseeded
    and diced
1 tbsp flaky sea salt
5 large free-range eggs
160g tin best-quality tuna, such
    as Ortiz, drained and flaked
30g black olives, pitted and halved
8–10 anchovy fillets in oil, drained
    and chopped
Vegetable oil, for cooking
25g butter
Sea salt and freshly ground
    black pepper

For the dressing:
1 small garlic clove, grated
½ tsp English mustard powder
1 tbsp chopped parsley
1 tbsp red wine vinegar
4 tbsp extra virgin olive oil

To finish (optional):
A handful of rocket leaves

1 In a bowl, mix together the cherry tomatoes, French beans, shallot, cucumber and flaky sea salt. Leave to stand for 15 minutes. Drain off any liquid from the salad vegetables and pat dry on kitchen paper.

2 Meanwhile, bring a saucepan of water to the boil, add one of the eggs and simmer for 7 minutes to hard-boil, then remove from the pan and cool under cold running water.

3 Mix the vegetables with the flaked tuna, olives and anchovies. Peel the hard-boiled egg and grate it into the mixture.

4 Whisk the remaining 4 eggs together in a bowl and season with salt and pepper.

5 For the dressing, whisk all the ingredients together in a small bowl. Set aside.

6 Warm a 24cm non-stick frying pan over a medium heat. Drizzle in a little oil and add the butter to the pan. When the butter is melted and stops foaming, pour in the egg and gently move it around until it sets. Try to cook the omelette all of the way through without letting it take on any colour. Gently slide the omelette out onto a plate.

7 Spoon the salad on top of the omelette and trickle over a few spoonfuls of the dressing. Finish with a scattering of rocket leaves if you like. Serve the rest of the dressing on the side.

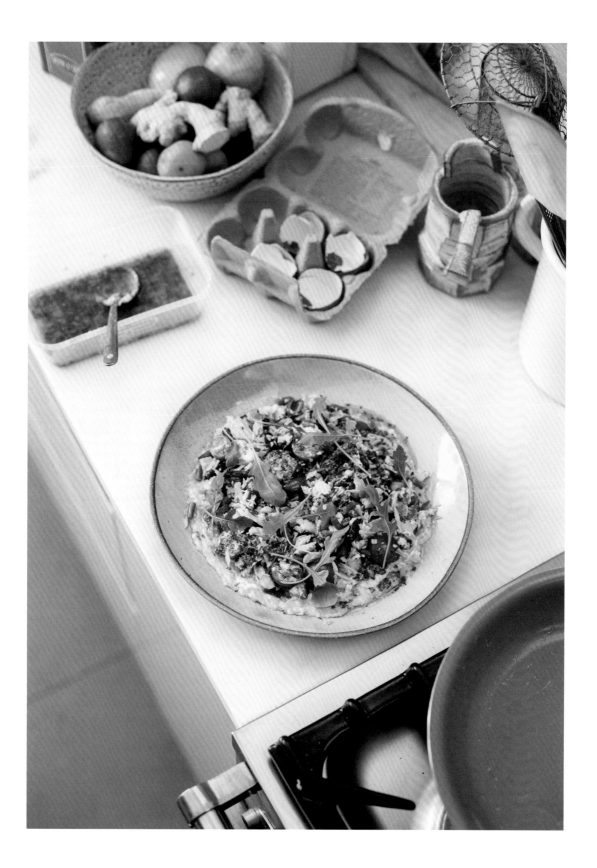

Lemon sole egg rolls with mushroom sauce

Even the most carb-hungry person will love this luxurious dish. If you can't get lemon sole, use another white fish such as bream, sea bass or plaice instead. Dried trompettes have a distinctive earthy, truffley flavour but you can use other dried mushrooms here, such as porcini. You can make your own mushroom powder if you like: simply blitz dried mushrooms in a small food processor to a fine powder. It keeps well, sealed in a container in a cool, dark cupboard.

Serves: 2

Carb count: 18g per person

20g dried trompette mushrooms

For the mushroom sauce:
30g butter
1 onion, finely diced
2 garlic cloves, grated
1 chicken stock cube
200ml double cream
175g large portobello mushrooms, diced
2 tbsp crème fraîche
Sea salt and freshly ground black pepper

For the egg rolls:
4 large free-range eggs
150g cream cheese
2 tsp dried mushroom powder
Vegetable oil, for cooking

To assemble:
30g butter
300g baby spinach
100g Gruyère cheese, grated
2 lemon soles, filleted, skinned (you can get your fishmonger to do this) and cut into 5cm goujons

1 Soak the dried mushrooms in 200ml boiling water for about 20 minutes. Tip into a muslin-lined sieve lined over a small bowl to drain off the soaking water; reserve this liquor. Roughly chop the soaked mushrooms.

2 To make the sauce, melt the butter in a large frying pan over a medium-low heat then add the onion and garlic. Sweat gently, stirring from time to time, for about 10–15 minutes until soft. Crumble in the stock cube and stir in the reserved mushroom liquor. Simmer until reduced to a glaze. Add the cream and diced portobello mushrooms, bring to a simmer and simmer gently for 5–8 minutes until the sauce thickens slightly. Remove from the heat and stir in the crème fraîche. Season with salt and pepper to taste and set aside.

3 Preheat the oven to 200°C/Fan 180°C/Gas 6. To make the egg rolls, whisk together the eggs, cream cheese and mushroom powder to make a light batter. Warm a 24cm non-stick frying pan over a medium heat. Drizzle in a little oil and then pour in a quarter of the batter. Fry until browned underneath then flip over and cook the other side. Remove and drain on kitchen paper; keep warm. Repeat with the rest of the mix to make 4 pancakes.

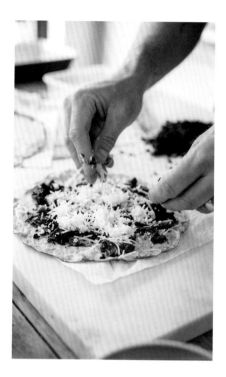

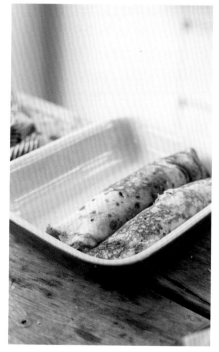

④ To assemble, warm the butter in a large frying pan over a medium heat, add the spinach and sweat until just wilted. Tip into a colander and drain. Squeeze out the liquid in a clean tea towel or using several layers of kitchen paper. Chop the spinach to a rough purée.

⑤ Cover each pancake with a generous spoonful of spinach. Scatter on some chopped soaked mushrooms, grated Gruyère and fish goujons, then top with more cheese. Roll the pancakes up, place them side by side in an ovenproof dish and pour on the mushroom sauce. Bake for 12–15 minutes, until golden and bubbling. Serve straight away.

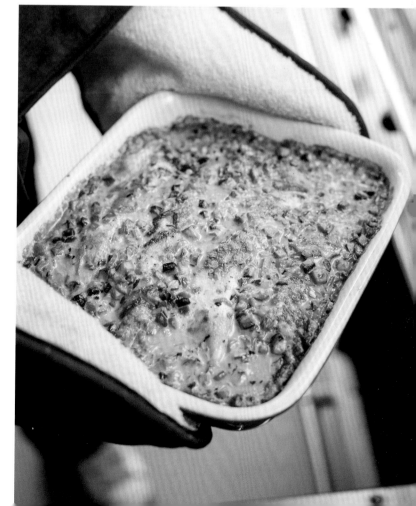

Salt cod, chorizo and saffron omelette

I love the combination of egg, chorizo, salt cod and saffron so much that it's been on the menu at The Hand and Flowers for a number of years – in the form of our popular Scotch egg. I thought it would be a good idea to bring the same Spanish assembly together in an easy, tasty omelette.

Serves: 2–4

Carb count: 21–11g per person

1 tbsp rock salt
½ tbsp caster sugar
2 pinches of saffron strands
75ml white wine
250g cod fillet, skinned and
    pin-boned
Extra virgin olive oil, to drizzle
3 chorizo sausages, for cooking
    (about 280g in total), cut into
    bite-sized chunks
6 large free-range eggs
1 tsp smoked paprika
3 tbsp chopped, jarred roasted
    red peppers
2 red chillies, sliced, seeds and all
100g Manchego cheese, grated
Sea salt and freshly ground
    black pepper

For the spinach salad:
150g baby spinach
1 banana shallot, thinly sliced
    into rings
1 tbsp capers
A trickle of extra virgin olive oil

1 Mix the rock salt and sugar with a pinch of saffron. Add half the wine and mix to a paste. Put the cod fillet into a bowl, cover with the cure and massage it into the fish. Cover the bowl with cling film and refrigerate for 1 hour. Rinse the fish under cold running water to remove the cure. Pat dry with kitchen paper.

2 Preheat the oven to 180°C/Fan 160°C/Gas 4. Lay the cod fillet on a large square of foil and drizzle over some olive oil. Wrap the fish in the foil and seal the edges to form a parcel. Lift into a roasting tin and bake in the oven for 25 minutes. Remove and set aside to cool in the foil.

3 In a small saucepan over a low heat, warm the remaining wine and saffron. Allow to infuse for a couple of minutes then take off the heat and set aside to cool.

4 Warm a 24cm non-stick ovenproof frying pan over a medium heat. Pour in a little olive oil and then add the pieces of chorizo. Fry gently, until the chorizo is cooked through and its lovely red oil is released into the pan.

5 Meanwhile, whisk the eggs with the saffron-infused wine, smoked paprika and some salt and pepper. Pour into the pan and stir gently over a low heat, until the egg just starts to set. Remove from the heat.

6 Flake the cooked cod on top of the egg. Scatter over the red peppers and chillies, then the grated cheese. Place the pan in the oven and cook for 12 minutes, until just set.

7 Meanwhile, for the salad, mix together the baby spinach, shallot, capers and olive oil. Season with salt and pepper to taste.

8 Remove the omelette from the oven and leave to stand in the pan for 3–4 minutes, then carefully slide it out onto a warm plate. Serve the spinach salad on the side.

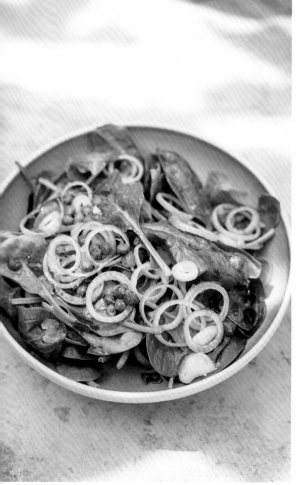

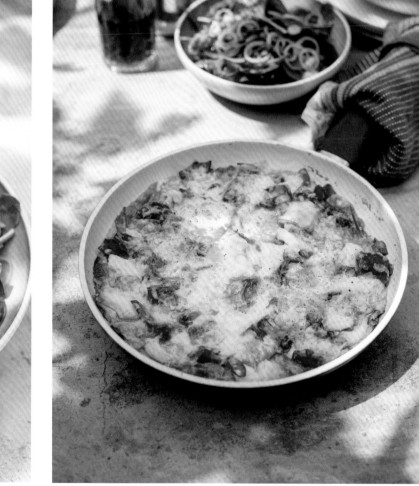

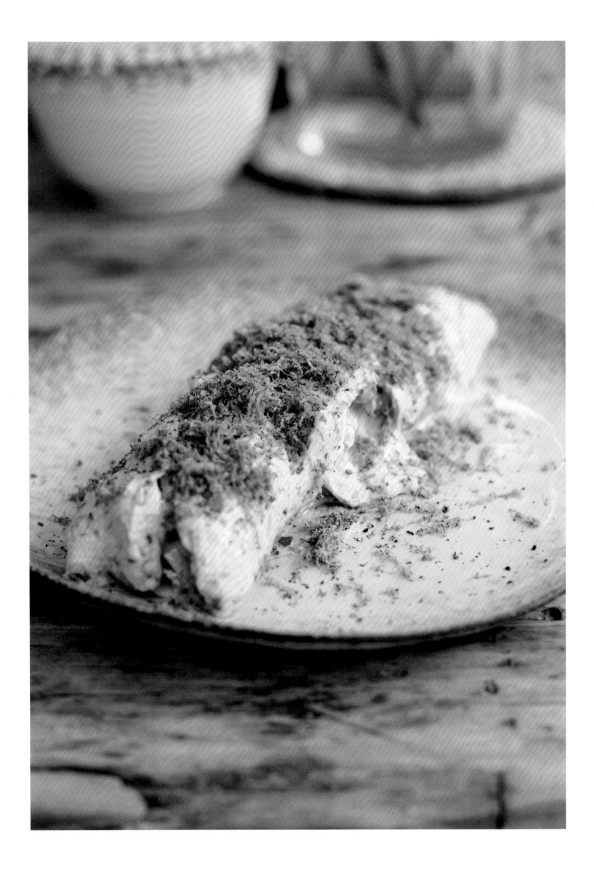

Chicken forestière omelette

Chicken forestière, a classic dish of chicken and mushrooms in a rich white wine sauce, features here as a delicious filling for a sustaining omelette. I often use leftover roast chicken for this, or you can simply cook a chicken breast before you get started. Grating over some black truffle at the end makes it extra special.

Serves: 2

Carb count: 10g per person

Vegetable oil, for cooking
1 onion, finely diced
2 garlic cloves, grated
1 chicken stock cube
150ml white wine
100ml double cream
100g button mushrooms, quartered
150g cooked free-range chicken,
    cut into bite-sized pieces
4 large free-range eggs
4 tbsp chopped parsley
25g butter
Sea salt and freshly ground
    black pepper
1 small black truffle, to finish
    (optional)

1 Heat a little oil in a frying pan over a medium-low heat. Add the onion with the garlic and a pinch of salt and sweat for 10–15 minutes, stirring occasionally, until softened. Crumble in the stock cube then pour in the wine and 50ml water. Bring to the boil and let bubble to reduce to a glaze.

2 Pour in the cream, add the mushrooms and turn the heat down. Cook at a low simmer for about 10 minutes until the mushrooms soften and release their liquor into the sauce.

3 Stir in the cooked chicken and continue to cook until the sauce is thickened and coats the chicken, with very little liquor left in the pan. Take the pan off the heat and season the filling with salt and pepper to taste.

4 In a bowl, whisk together the eggs, chopped parsley and some salt and pepper.

5 Heat a non-stick frying pan over a low heat and add the butter. When it stops foaming, pour in the egg mix and gently move it around in the pan until the omelette is set.

6 Spoon the chicken and mushroom mixture into the middle of the omelette and roll up. Place on a warmed plate and grate over some black truffle, if you have one. Cut the omelette in half to serve.

Sausage, sage and onion omelette

This is a simple play on the nation's favourite breakfast, or a twist on a sausage sandwich. Whichever way you see it, it makes a great lunch or quick supper, or a top-notch weekend breakfast.

Serves: 2

Carb count: 20g per person

6 best-quality sausages, cooked, cooled and chilled
Vegetable oil, for cooking
25g butter
2 onions, finely diced
2 garlic cloves, grated
4 large free-range eggs
2 tbsp English mustard
2 tbsp chopped sage leaves
Sea salt and freshly ground black pepper

1 Preheat the oven to 200°C/Fan 180°C/Gas 6. Cut the sausages into bite-sized pieces. Warm a 24cm non-stick ovenproof frying pan over a medium heat. Drizzle in some oil and fry the sausage pieces until browned and crisp around the edges. Remove from the pan and drain on kitchen paper.

2 Add the butter to the pan and, once it has melted, tip in the onions and garlic. Season with salt and pepper and sweat gently, stirring from time to time, until soft. This will take about 10–15 minutes.

3 Meanwhile, in a bowl, whisk the eggs with the mustard and some salt and pepper.

4 Pour the egg mixture into the pan and cook just until the bottom begins to set. Add the cooked sausage and chopped sage, then place the pan in the oven for 10–12 minutes, until the egg is just set on top.

5 Leave to stand for 3–4 minutes then slide the omelette out onto a plate. Serve some crisp-grilled bacon rashers on the side if you like.

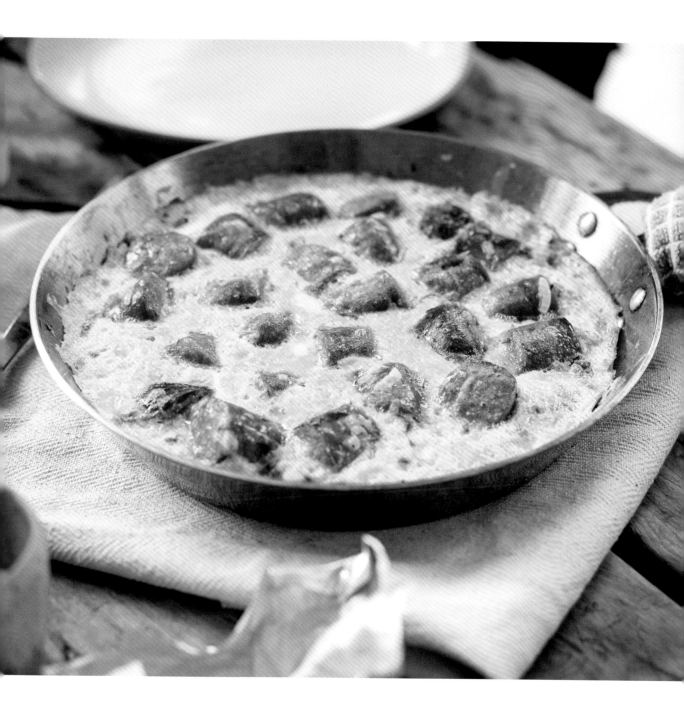

Ham hock, kale and Cheddar omelette

This works beautifully as a classy, French rolled omelette. It looks great, but it's very simple to make. I really like the robust, minerally flavour of the kale with the rich egg and crispy ham hock. Serve it as it is, or with a crisp green salad.

Serves: 2	
Carb count: 2g per person	

150g kale, tough stems removed, torn into even-sized pieces
Vegetable oil, for cooking
90g packet of cooked flaked ham hock
1 large garlic clove, grated
6 large free-range eggs
25g butter
75g mature Cheddar cheese, grated
Sea salt and freshly ground black pepper

1 Put a bowl of iced water next to the hob. Bring a pan of salted water to the boil. Add the kale and blanch for 3–4 minutes, until it softens. Drain and refresh in the iced water. Once cooled, drain and squeeze out as much excess water as possible, using a clean tea towel or kitchen paper. Roughly chop the kale and set aside.

2 Heat a little oil in a non-stick frying pan over a medium-high heat and fry the ham hock until browned and crispy. Add the garlic and cook for a further minute. Drain the ham hock on some kitchen paper.

3 Turn the heat under the frying pan down to low and give it a quick wipe out with a wad of kitchen paper.

4 Whisk the eggs together in a bowl and season with salt and pepper.

5 Melt the butter in the frying pan and then pour in the beaten egg. Keep moving the egg around gently so that it cooks without taking on any colour.

6 When the omelette is almost cooked through, scatter over the kale, crispy ham and grated cheese. Roll the omelette up and serve it immediately, with a crisp green salad on the side if you fancy.

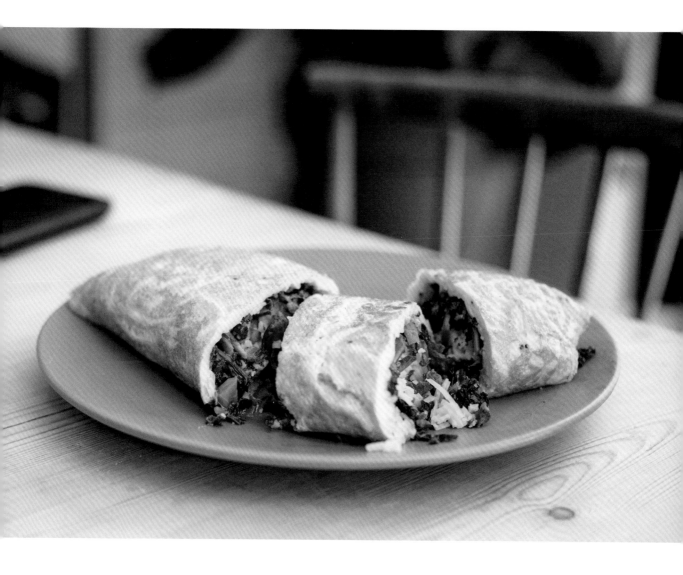

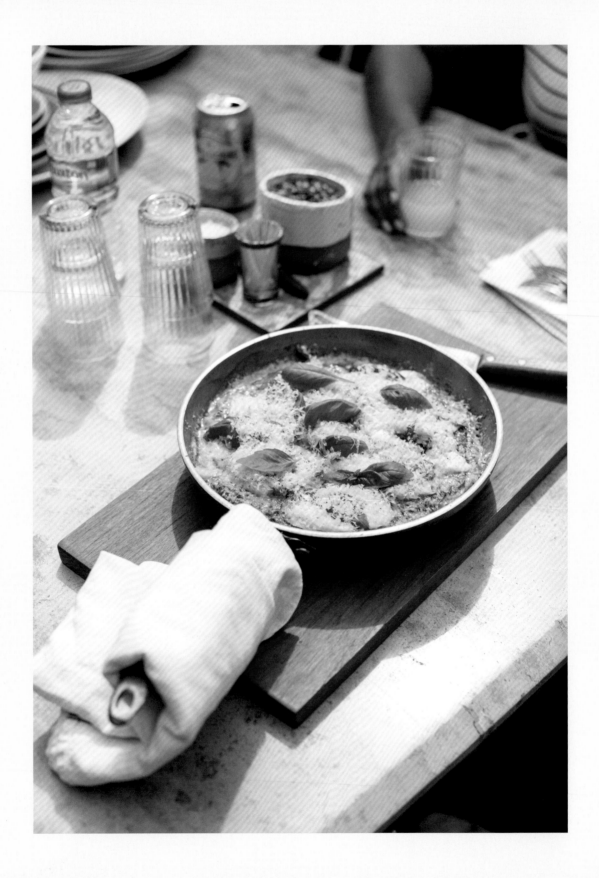

Pepperoni pizza omelette

This has all the flavours of a great pizza but without the heavy carbs. How lush is that? It's just the sort of thing I love when I'm hungry and in a hurry, as I can make it from the sort of ingredients I almost always have to hand. Feel free to swap the pepperoni for slices of chorizo or any other favourite cured, sliced sausage.

Serves: 2–4

Carb count: 16–8g per person

250ml passata
2 tbsp tomato purée
3 garlic cloves, grated
6 large free-range eggs
2 tsp dried oregano
A drizzle of olive oil
150g sliced pepperoni
2 balls of mozzarella (about
    125g each), drained
2 tbsp fresh oregano leaves
30g Parmesan cheese
A small handful of basil leaves
Sea salt and freshly ground
    black pepper

1 To make the tomato sauce, heat the passata, tomato purée and garlic in a saucepan over a medium heat. Simmer to reduce until the sauce is nice and thick. This will take about 8–10 minutes. Remove from the heat, season with salt and pepper to taste and leave to cool.

2 Preheat the oven to 200°C/Fan 180°C/Gas 6. In a bowl, whisk together the eggs and dried oregano and season with salt and pepper.

3 Heat a little olive oil in a 24cm non-stick ovenproof frying pan over a medium-high heat. Pour in the egg and stir until it is almost fully cooked, removing the pan from the heat when the omelette is still a little runny and wobbly in the middle.

4 Gently spread the tomato sauce all over the omelette. Cover with the pepperoni, then tear the mozzarella into pieces and scatter it over.

5 Sprinkle with the oregano and then place the pan in the oven for 8–10 minutes, until the cheese has melted and the 'pizza' is set.

6 Remove from the oven and immediately grate the Parmesan over the top. Scatter over the basil and serve at once, directly from the pan.

Quattro stagioni omelette

I've transported all the great, quattro stagioni pizza toppings onto an omelette and the results are pretty good! The big, strong flavours of black olives, marinated artichokes, mushrooms and salty ham make this a very satisfying dish.

Serves: 2–4

Carb count: 28–14g per person

250ml passata
2 tbsp tomato purée
4 garlic cloves, grated
6 large free-range eggs
1 tbsp dried herbes de Provence
Extra virgin olive oil, to trickle
25g butter
A large handful of black olives
   (about 100g), pitted
4 slices of Parma ham
8 baby artichokes preserved in oil,
   halved lengthways
200g button mushrooms, quartered
2 balls of mozzarella (about
   125g each), drained
2 tbsp oregano or basil leaves
Sea salt and freshly ground
   black pepper

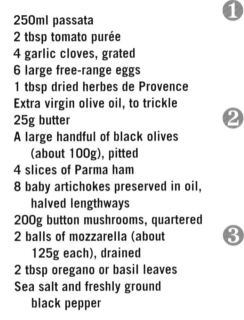

The Dope: Artichokes preserved in oil are a great store-cupboard standby. Include them in salads and antipasti, or to make a 'pizza omelette' topping.

1 To make the tomato sauce, warm the passata, tomato purée and garlic in a saucepan over a medium heat. Simmer to reduce until the sauce is nice and thick; this will take about 8–10 minutes. Remove from the heat, season with salt and pepper to taste and leave to cool.

2 Preheat the oven to 200°C/Fan 180°C/Gas 6. In a bowl, whisk the eggs together with the dried herbs and some salt and pepper.

3 Heat a little oil in a 24cm non-stick ovenproof frying pan over a medium-high heat. Add the butter and, when it has melted and stopped foaming, pour in the egg. Stir until it is almost fully cooked, removing the pan from the heat when the omelette is still a little runny and wobbly in the middle.

4 Gently spread the tomato sauce all over the omelette. Arrange the olives over one quarter, the ham in another quarter, then place the artichokes in the third quarter. Fill the last quarter of the 'pizza' with the mushrooms. Trickle over some olive oil.

5 Roughly tear the mozzarella and scatter it over the top. Place the pan in the oven for 10–12 minutes, until the cheese has melted and the egg is fully set. Remove the omelette from the oven and scatter over the oregano or basil leaves. Grind over some pepper and serve immediately, straight from the pan.

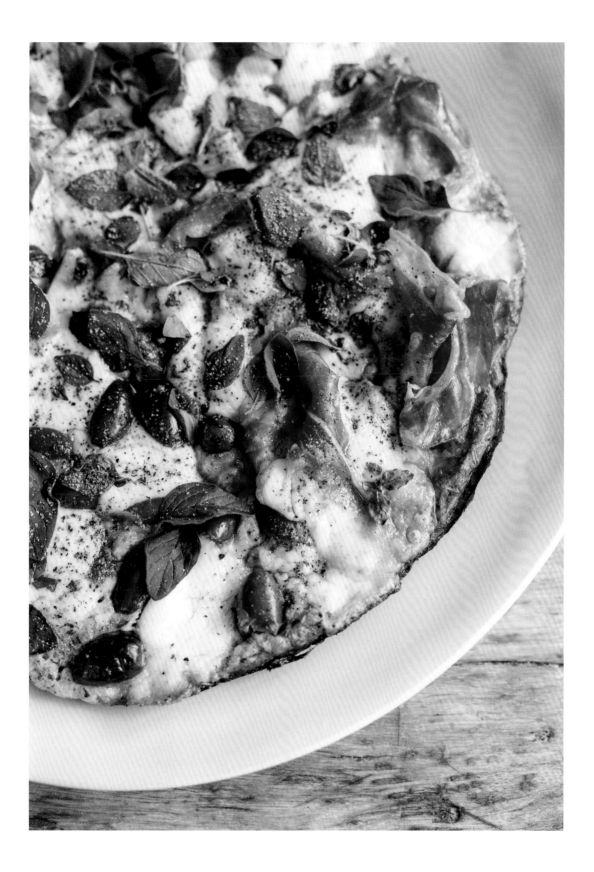

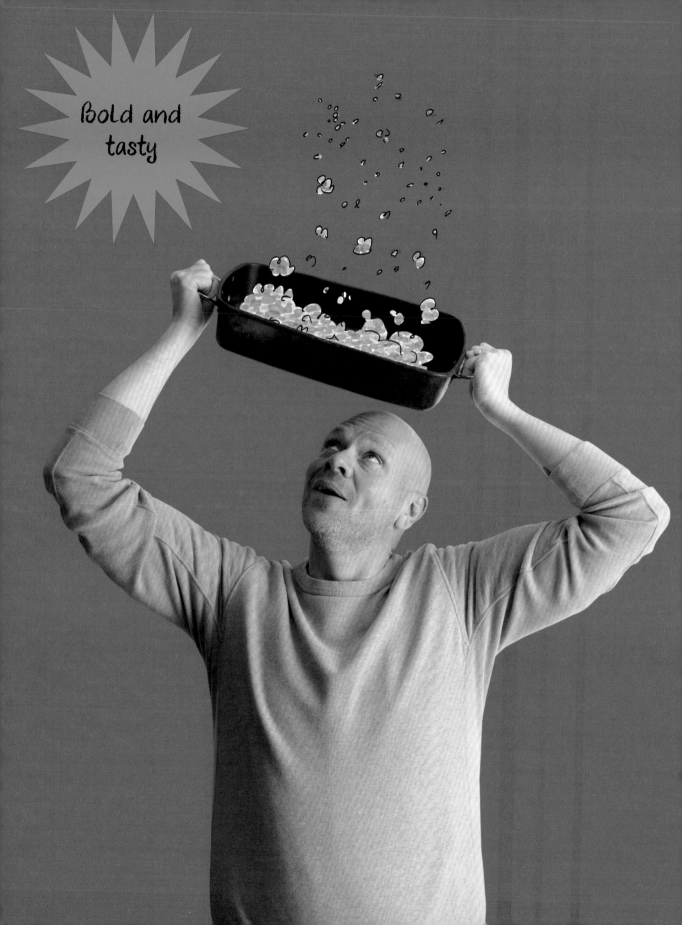

MINCED MEAT DISHES

REALISE IT'S RARE for a Michelin-starred chef to get really excited by mince, but I love it! It's one of those things we all grew up eating as a weekly staple – as burgers, bolognese sauce, chilli, pies or meatloaf.

When I started putting together the recipes for this book, I decided to use everyday ingredients – the kind of things you might pick up in your weekly shop – and turn them into something really fantastic, to give you new ideas that will help you feel satisfied and happy as you embark on this new way of eating.

There are few foods more versatile than mince. It suffers from 'Cinderella syndrome', overlooked in favour of flashy, more expensive cuts. Everyone is impressed by fillet of beef or a lovely loin of pork and it can be easy to forget that mince comes from the very same beasts. If it's a beautiful, well-reared animal, why should we be any less excited about mince? It will still be fantastic quality. If you embrace mince with the same love as you do the more pricey cuts, you'll definitely get a lot more out of it in the end.

A technique at the heart of so many of the dishes in this chapter is roasting the mince before you start. This is something that many cooks – even very good cooks – have never tried before. I promise you it's worth that bit of extra effort as it lifts the flavour and texture of the finished dish to another level. It needn't be a massive chore. You don't have to do very much – simply bung the mince in the oven or in a pan on the hob and roast it, giving it a good stir now and again, until it's a rich golden brown. If it suits you better, you can even do this the day before and keep the browned mince in the fridge until you're ready. Try it once and I promise you'll be converted. It will help you make bolognese (see page 150), shepherd's pie (see page 138) and chilli (see page 144) that are truly tasty.

Along with the benefit to the flavour, I can't begin to say enough about what pre-roasting mince does to its texture. When you're on any kind of diet, one of the things you miss the most is crunchy, chewy texture – that sense of really getting your teeth into something. Try my crispy vinegar pork with cauliflower purée (page 156), for example. Silky cauliflower is paired with chewy little nuggets of meat which are packed with flavour – it's completely satisfying.

Mince takes on all kinds of seasonings beautifully, whether it's Mediterranean herbs or Asian spices, whether you want to create something cosy and comforting or exciting and exotic. You'll also find plenty of ingredients that can help boost dopamine levels in these mince dishes, including low-carb vegetables such as cauliflower, turnips and kohlrabi. Rich and layered with great flavours, beautifully cooked mince is delicious.

The recipes that follow represent something I believe in wholeheartedly, that you can take fairly humble ingredients and – with a bit of care and knowledge – transform them into something quite outstanding. If you're just going to have a bowl of mince, why shouldn't it be the best, most luxurious bowl of mince you've ever tasted?

Buy good-quality mince

If at all possible, get your mince from a decent butcher. That way, if you're buying it straight from their chiller, you'll have some confidence about what's in it. Or you can have them grind up specific cuts to get just the flavour, texture and fat content you want. The difference between cheap mince and the good stuff is quite dramatic, so it's worth taking a bit of extra trouble.

Chicken and coconut curry

This curry is so rich and indulgent, I love tucking into a bowl of it and I really don't miss the carby rice or bread at all. I use chicken mince here, made from the thigh meat, which is moist and full of flavour. A good butcher should be happy to mince chicken thighs for you.

Serves: 4

Carb count: 15g per person

Vegetable oil, for cooking
1kg minced free-range chicken
    thigh meat
2 onions, finely diced
8 garlic cloves, grated
4cm knob of fresh ginger, grated
2 tsp salt
1 tsp ground ginger
1 tsp ground turmeric
1 tsp ground cumin
1 tsp ground cinnamon
1 tsp chilli powder
400ml tin coconut milk
½ x 400g tin chopped tomatoes
50g desiccated coconut, toasted
    in a dry frying pan until golden
    and fragrant
2 hot green chillies, thinly sliced,
    seeds and all
Juice of 1 lemon
6 tbsp freshly chopped coriander,
    tender stems and all
4 tbsp chopped pickled green
    chillies
Sea salt and freshly ground
    black pepper

1 Heat a large saucepan over a medium-high heat, pour in a little oil and then add the chicken. Cook, stirring frequently, until it is almost dry, lightly browned and crumbly. This will take at least 20–25 minutes. Tip the mince into a colander and leave to drain.

2 Return the pan to the heat and pour in a little more oil. Add the onions and cook over a medium heat until softened and starting to colour, about 10–15 minutes. Add the garlic and cook, stirring, for a further 4–5 minutes until the onions take on a little more of a golden colour. Add the grated ginger, salt and all of the dry spices. Stir and cook for 2–3 minutes until very fragrant.

3 Return the browned mince to the pan, pour in the coconut milk and stir in the chopped tomatoes. Bring to the boil, then turn down the heat and simmer for 10–15 minutes, until the sauce has thickened slightly (don't worry if it looks split).

4 Stir in the toasted coconut and fresh chillies and cook for 3–4 minutes, until the curry thickens. Season with the lemon juice, salt and pepper then stir in the chopped coriander and pickled chillies. Serve in warmed bowls.

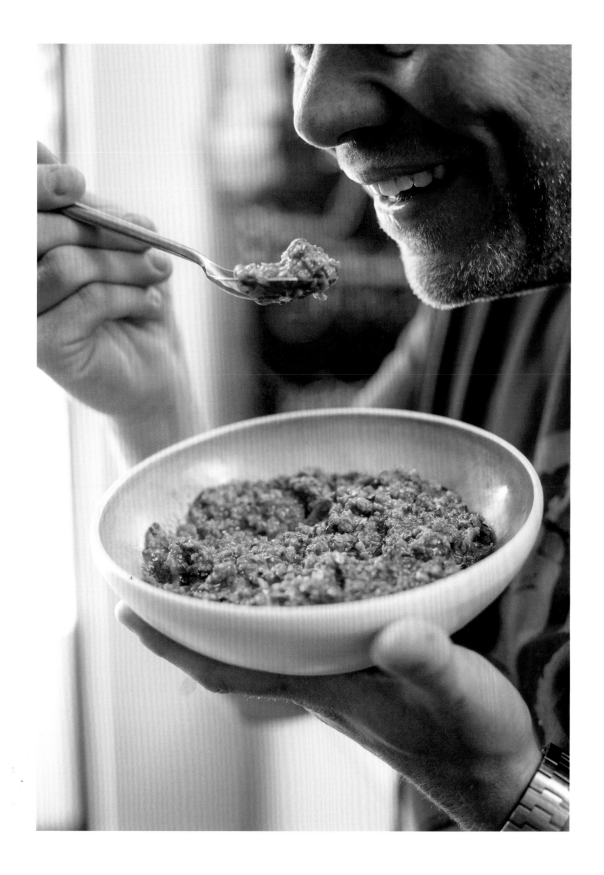

Turkey burgers with kohlrabi slaw

For burgers, turkey is an excellent alternative to beef or pork and it takes on seasonings beautifully. It's great with the sage and spices here. These burgers are easy to make and just as good for a weeknight tea or a summer barbecue. I love the flavour and crunch of coleslaw and this is one of the simplest and best.

Serves: 4

Carb count: 8g per person

For the turkey burgers:
800g minced turkey
200g sausage meat
2 tsp salt
2 tsp dried sage
2 tsp dried chilli flakes
1 tsp cayenne pepper
1 tsp garlic powder
1 tsp cracked black pepper
Vegetable oil, for cooking
4 slices of strong Cheddar cheese

For the kohlrabi slaw:
2 kohlrabi, peeled and cut into
**   julienne**
1 onion, halved and thinly sliced
2 tsp flaky sea salt
2 tbsp thick mayonnaise
1 tbsp wholegrain mustard
A bunch of chives (about 20g),
**   finely chopped**

To serve:
Pickled green chillies
Favourite condiments, such as
**   mustard, mayonnaise and/or**
**   Sriracha sauce**

1 To make the burgers, put the turkey, sausage meat, salt, sage, chilli flakes, cayenne pepper, garlic powder and black pepper into a bowl. Work the ingredients together to combine, using your hands, then knead the mixture as you would bread, until it firms up.

2 Dampen your hands a little with cold water. Divide the mixture into 4 portions and form each into a ball, then flatten slightly to make burgers. Place on a plate, cover with cling film and refrigerate for at least 1 hour to rest. You can make the burgers up to 24 hours ahead and keep them refrigerated.

3 Meanwhile, make the slaw. In a large bowl, mix the kohlrabi julienne, onion and flaky salt together and leave to stand for 10 minutes. Tip into a colander and rinse under cold, running water. Pat dry on a clean tea towel or with kitchen paper. Place in a clean bowl and stir in the mayonnaise and mustard, then fold in the chives.

4 Heat a little oil in a non-stick frying pan over a medium-high heat and cook the burgers for about 5–6 minutes each side until cooked through. Or you can grill or barbecue them: first rub the surface of the burgers with a little oil to stop them sticking, then cook for about 12 minutes, turning 2–3 times.

Lay a slice of Cheddar on top of each burger and place under a hot grill until the cheese has melted.

 Serve the turkey burgers with the kohlrabi slaw, pickled green chillies, your favourite condiments and any tasty salad you fancy.

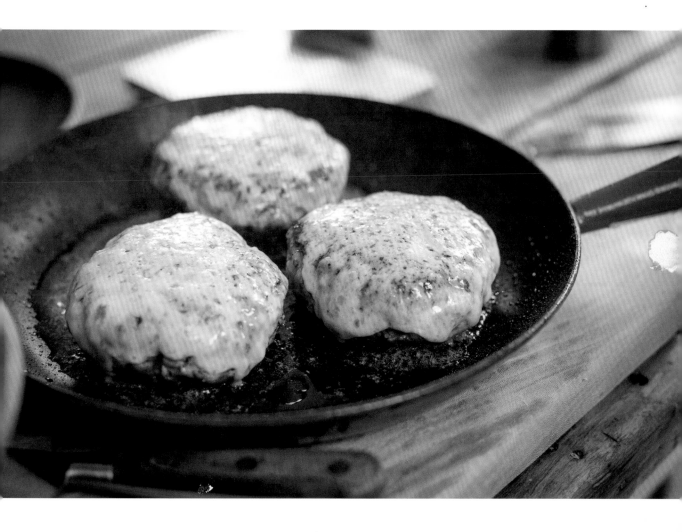

Moussaka

There are few dishes more comforting than this cosy classic. With its tasty meat ragu, layered with aubergines and topped with a rich cheesy custard, it's a great dinner for a cold evening. It takes a little while to put together, but every step is easy so don't be put off from giving it a go.

Serves: 6

Carb count: 16g per person

1kg good-quality minced lamb
Olive oil, for cooking
1 onion, finely diced
3 garlic cloves, grated
2 tsp dried oregano
2 tsp ground cinnamon
2 tsp dried mint
2 tsp cracked black pepper
2 tbsp tomato purée
500ml beef stock
400g tin chopped tomatoes
2 green chillies, finely diced, seeds and all
3 large aubergines
Sea salt and freshly ground black pepper

For the topping:
4 free-range eggs, plus an extra 2 egg yolks
500ml double cream
½ tsp ground cumin
½ tsp ground cinnamon
150g Gruyère cheese, grated
100g Parmesan cheese, freshly grated

1 Preheat the oven to 200°C/Fan 180°C/Gas 6. Place the lamb mince in a large roasting tin and roast for 30–35 minutes, stirring a few times to break it up, until roasted and dark brown. It should look like instant coffee granules. You can also do this in a large frying pan on the hob if you like – just make sure you get it good and dark. Tip the mince into a colander and set aside to drain.

2 Warm a splash of olive oil in a large saucepan over a medium-low heat. Add the onion and garlic and sauté gently for 10–15 minutes until soft, stirring from time to time. Add the oregano, cinnamon, dried mint and cracked black pepper. Cook, stirring, for 2–3 minutes. Add the tomato purée and cook for a further 3–4 minutes.

3 Tip the drained mince into the saucepan and add the stock and tinned tomatoes. Bring to the boil then turn down the heat. Simmer, uncovered, until the sauce is reduced and thickened to a rich ragu, stirring occasionally and checking that it isn't sticking to the bottom of the pan or drying out. This should take about an hour. Add the diced chillies, remove from the heat and season with salt and pepper to taste.

Continues overleaf ➔

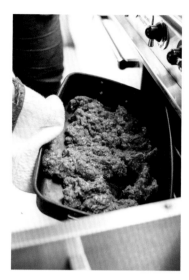

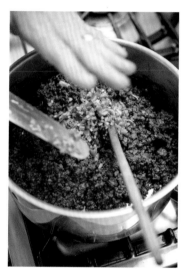

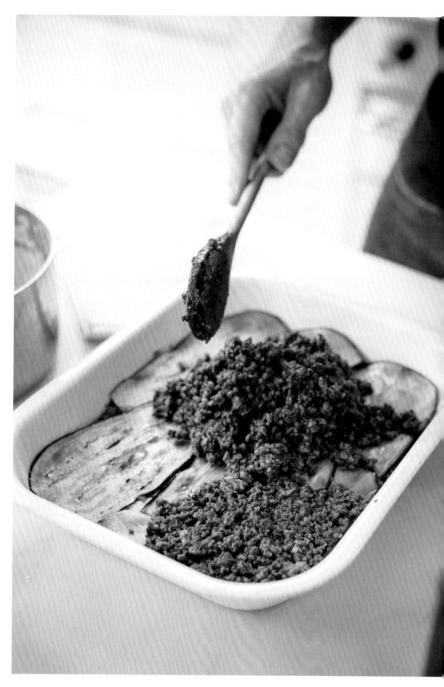

Continued from previous page →

④ Meanwhile, prepare the aubergines. Slice them lengthways as thinly as you can, about 4mm thick. Sprinkle the slices with salt, lay on kitchen paper and leave to stand for 10–15 minutes until softened. Rinse under cold running water, then pat dry on a clean tea towel or with kitchen paper.

⑤ Heat some olive oil in a large frying pan over a medium-high heat and fry the aubergine slices until golden on both sides. You'll need to do this in batches. Drain on kitchen paper.

⑥ Preheat the oven to 180°C/Fan 160°C/Gas 4. Spoon a third of the lamb ragu into a shallow ovenproof dish, about 32 x 22cm and 8cm deep. Place a layer of cooked aubergines on top, then repeat these layers twice more, ending with an aubergine layer.

⑦ To make the topping, whisk the whole eggs and egg yolks together in a large bowl. Pour the cream into a saucepan and stir in the cumin and cinnamon. Bring to a simmer, then pour onto the eggs, whisking as you do so. Pour through a sieve back into the pan and warm gently, stirring, until it thickens. Stir in the grated cheeses and take off the heat. Season with salt and pepper to taste.

⑧ Pour the rich, savoury custard on top of the moussaka. Stand the dish on a baking tray and bake in the oven for 25–30 minutes until the topping has set. Now brown briefly under a hot grill or using a cook's blowtorch. Leave the moussaka to stand for 5 minutes or so before serving. Serve with a crisp green salad if you like.

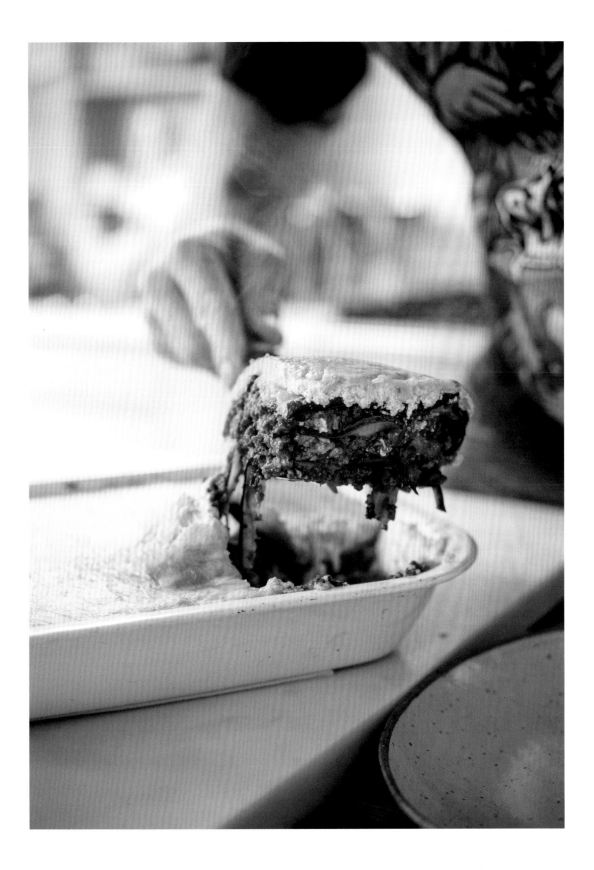

Lamb ragu, courgette spaghetti, feta and mint

This is such a great, tasty dish. The powerful flavours of the ragu combine so beautifully with the subtle, smooth courgette spaghetti – and everyone knows lamb, feta and mint is a winner.

Serves: 4–6
Carb count: 27–18g per person

1kg good-quality minced lamb
Olive oil, for cooking
2 onions, finely diced
4 garlic cloves, grated
2 tbsp tomato purée
1 tbsp cumin seeds
75ml white wine vinegar
30g demerara sugar
200ml white wine
500ml lamb or beef stock
150g portobello mushrooms, diced
3 green chillies, diced, seeds and all
4 medium courgettes (about 500g in total)
75g butter
200g feta cheese, crumbled
A bunch of mint (about 25g), tough stems removed and leaves chopped
Sea salt and freshly ground black pepper

1 Preheat the oven to 200°C/Fan 180°C/Gas 6. Place the lamb mince in a large roasting tin and roast, stirring 3 or 4 times to break up the mince, for 35–40 minutes until roasted and dark brown. It should look like instant coffee granules. Tip the mince into a colander to drain.

2 Warm a splash of olive oil in a large frying pan over a medium-low heat, add the onions and garlic and sauté gently, stirring from time to time, for 10–15 minutes until softened. Add the tomato purée and cumin seeds and cook, stirring occasionally, for 4–5 minutes.

3 Add the browned mince, wine vinegar and demerara sugar to the pan and stir to mix. Turn the heat up a bit, bring to the boil and then pour in the wine. Let the liquor bubble and reduce down to a glaze. Pour in the stock, stir and bring to the boil.

4 Add the diced mushrooms, turn the heat down to a simmer and cook, uncovered, for 45 minutes–1 hour, or until the sauce has thickened to a rich ragu. Remove from the heat and stir in the green chillies. Season with salt and pepper to taste.

5 Around 10 minutes before you want to eat, put the courgettes through a spiralizer to turn them into thin 'spaghetti'.

6 Melt the butter in a saucepan. Add about 100ml water and some salt and pepper. Bring to the boil, then drop in the courgette spaghetti and turn it around for 1–2 minutes until it is slightly softened; don't overcook – you want it still to have some bite.

7 Fork the crumbled feta and chopped mint through the wilted courgettes and divide between warmed plates. Spoon the lamb ragu on top and serve.

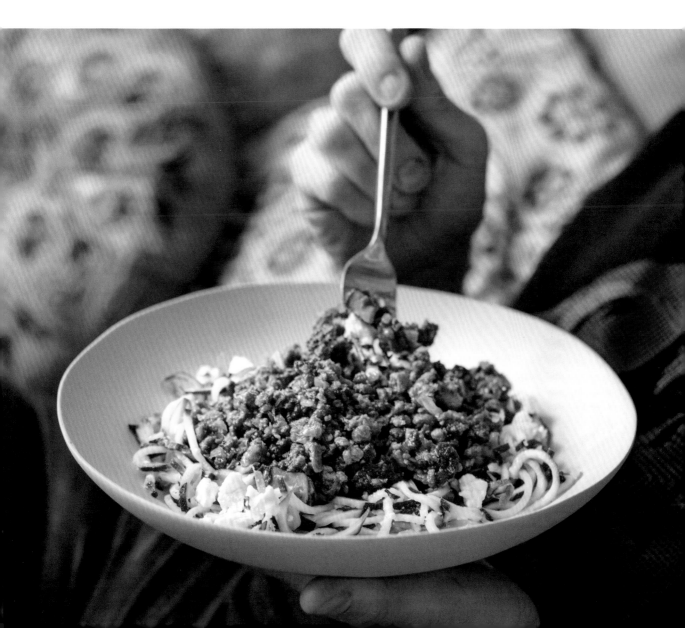

Shepherd's pie with creamy cauliflower topping

There are lots of big flavours in this not-quite-so-classic comfort food dinner. With spicy merguez sausages simmered with the lamb and a creamy cauliflower purée topping enriched with tangy blue cheese, it really hits the spot – and doesn't taste anything like diet food! Also, you can prepare it ahead, ready to bake and serve.

Serves: 6
Carb count: 22g per person

800g good-quality minced lamb
8 merguez sausages
Vegetable oil, for cooking
2 onions, diced
4 garlic cloves, grated
1 tbsp fennel seeds
2 tsp curry powder
2 tsp cracked black pepper
1 tsp ground cinnamon
4 celery sticks, tough strings
    removed, diced
500ml strong beef stock
A good dash of Worcestershire
    sauce
Sea salt and freshly ground
    black pepper

For the topping:
2 cauliflowers (about 700g each),
    cut into large florets
50g butter, softened
70ml double cream
200g strong blue cheese, such
    as Stilton, crumbled

1 Preheat the oven to 200°C/Fan 180°C/Gas 6. Place the lamb mince in a large roasting tin and roast, stirring 3 or 4 times to break up the mince, for 35–40 minutes until dark brown. It should look like instant coffee granules. Bake the merguez sausages in another roasting tin, alongside the lamb, for 10–15 minutes until cooked through.

2 Tip the mince into a colander to drain. Let the sausages cool, then cut into chunks.

3 Pour a splash of oil into a large saucepan and warm over a medium-low heat. Add the onions and garlic and sweat gently, stirring from time to time, for 10–15 minutes until soft. Stir in the fennel seeds, curry powder, cracked pepper and cinnamon and cook, stirring, for 2–3 minutes.

4 Stir in the celery and browned mince. Pour in the stock and add the Worcestershire sauce and some salt. Bring to the boil, lower the heat and simmer for 1–1½ hours, until beautifully thick and rich. Take off the heat and allow to cool.

5 Preheat the oven to 190°C/Fan 170°C/Gas 5. Stir the chopped sausages into the cooled lamb, then spoon into a shallow ovenproof dish, about 30 x 22cm and 8cm deep. Level the surface with the back of the spoon.

For the topping, bring a pan of lightly salted water to the boil, add the cauliflower florets and simmer until tender, about 5 minutes.

6 Drain the cauliflower and place in a food processor with the butter, cream and some salt and pepper. Blend until smooth. Add the blue cheese and blitz to combine.

Spoon the cauliflower topping evenly over the lamb and sausage mixture. Stand the dish on an oven tray and bake in the oven

7 for 30–35 minutes until the meat mixture is bubbling and the topping is starting to brown. Serve immediately.

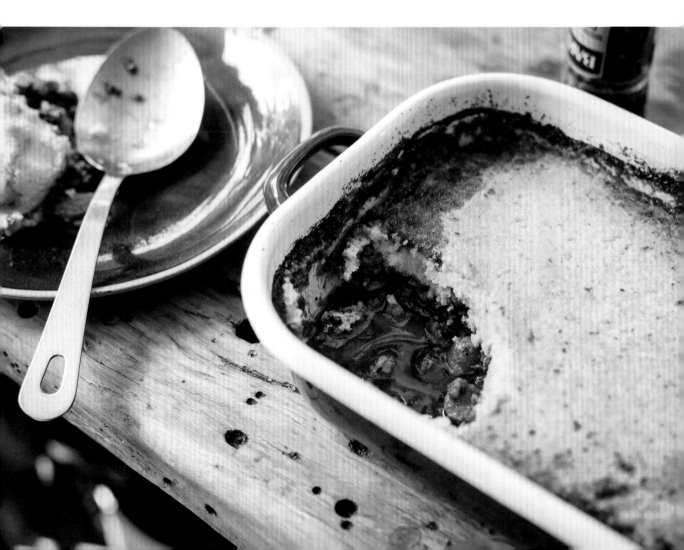

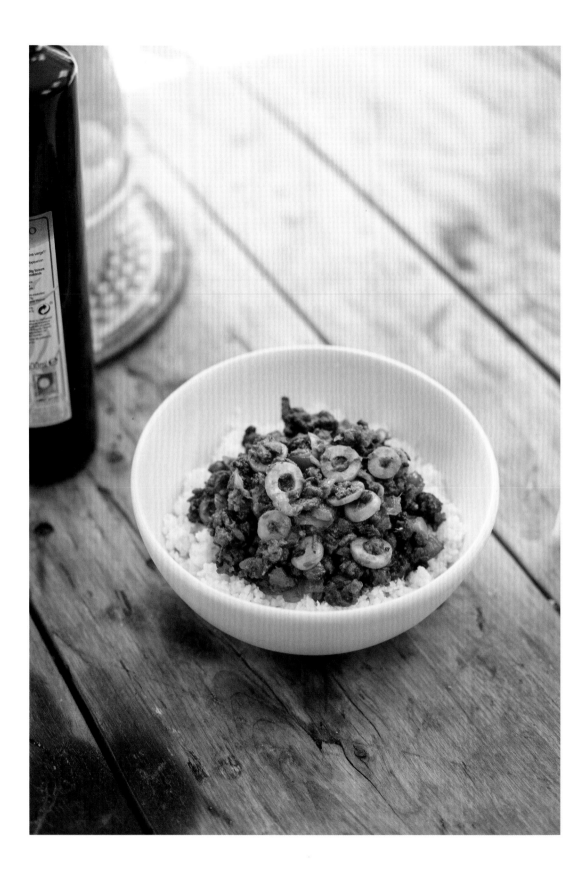

Cuban picadillo

This is a classic Cuban dish, usually eaten with black beans and rice, but since I've been on my low-carb kick I like it with cauliflower 'couscous' instead. You may notice I've omitted the dried fruit (typically raisins) included in a traditional picadillo – that's because it has too much sugar for my new regime.

Serves: 4–5

Carb count: 15–12g per person

750g best-quality minced beef
2 tbsp cumin seeds
1 tsp cracked black pepper
1 tsp garlic powder
1 tsp ground coriander
1 tsp dried oregano
1 tsp dried coriander leaf
1 tsp smoked paprika
1 tsp erythritol (sugar replacement)
1 tsp salt
A pinch of saffron strands
Vegetable oil, for cooking
2 onions, diced
4 garlic cloves, grated
1 green pepper, cored, deseeded
   and diced
2 beef stock cubes
450ml passata
150g green olives, pitted
   and sliced
3 tbsp capers

To serve (optional):
Cauliflower couscous (page 166)

1 Preheat the oven to 190°C/Fan 170°C/Gas 5. Put the mince in a roasting tin and roast for about 40 minutes, turning every 10 minutes or so, to get a very dark, even colour all over the meat. It should be crispy and resemble instant coffee granules. You can colour the meat in a large frying pan on the hob if you prefer; just keep stirring until it is dark brown. Drain in a colander and set aside.

2 In a small bowl, mix together the cumin seeds, cracked black pepper, garlic powder, ground coriander, dried oregano, dried coriander leaf, smoked paprika, erythritol, salt and saffron.

3 Heat up a large saucepan over a medium heat. Add a little oil, then the onions and garlic. Sweat gently, stirring from time to time, for 10–15 minutes until softened. Add the seasoning mix, stir and cook for 2–3 minutes.

4 Return the crispy beef to the pan and add the green pepper. Crumble in the stock cubes and pour on the passata. Bring to the boil, turn down the heat to a simmer and cook for 5–10 minutes until the sauce has thickened and is quite rich.

5 Add the olives and capers, stir, then check the seasoning and add more salt and pepper if required. Serve with the cauliflower couscous.

141

White radish lasagne

Trust me, this is a delicious, fail-safe recipe, which even die-hard carb lovers will love. The rich ragu is much as you would expect, but the 'pasta' layer is made from peppery white radish. You still get those great layers of texture and the melting cheese that you'd expect from any good lasagne. It takes a while to prepare, but none of the stages are difficult.

Serves: 6

Carb count: 23g per person

For the ragu:
800g best-quality minced beef
Vegetable oil, for cooking
250g bacon lardons, diced
2 tbsp caraway seeds
2 onions, diced
6 garlic cloves, grated
3 tbsp tomato purée
2 celery sticks, tough strings
   removed, diced
2 carrots, diced
2 tbsp dried herbes de Provence
500ml beef stock
400g tin chopped tomatoes
300ml red wine
250g button mushrooms, stalks
   removed, caps halved
2 tbsp chopped sage
Sea salt and freshly ground
   black pepper

To assemble:
2 large white radishes, also
   known as mooli or daikon
   (about 330g each)
3 balls of mozzarella (about 125g
   each), drained and torn into
   small pieces
200g Cheddar cheese, grated
200g crème fraîche

1 Preheat the oven to 190°C/Fan 170°C/Gas 5. Put the mince in a roasting tin and roast for about 40 minutes, turning every 10 minutes or so, to get a very dark, even colour all over the meat. It should be crispy and resemble instant coffee granules. You can colour the meat in a large frying pan on the hob if you prefer; just keep stirring until it is dark brown. Drain in a colander and set aside.

2 Warm a splash of oil in a large saucepan over a medium heat. Add the lardons and cook, stirring from time to time, until they have rendered some of their fat and started to brown. Lift them out of the pan with a slotted spoon and tip into the colander with the beef mince. Reserve the fat in the pan.

3 Toss the caraway seeds into the pan and toast for 2–3 minutes until fragrant. Add the onions and garlic and sweat gently, stirring from time to time, for 10–15 minutes until softened. Add the tomato purée and cook, stirring, for 3–4 minutes. Tip in the celery, carrots and dried herbs. Stir and cook for 5 minutes.

4 Return the beef and bacon to the pan and pour in the stock, tinned tomatoes and wine. Bring to the boil, reduce the heat to a simmer

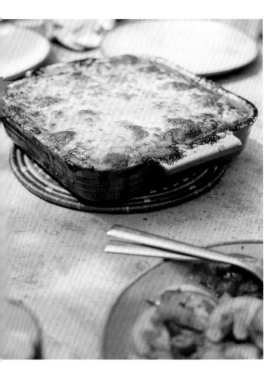

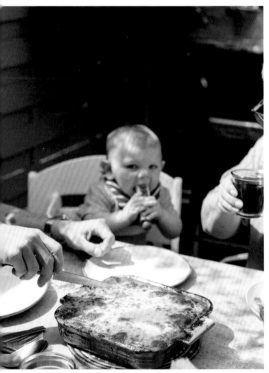

and stir in the mushrooms. Cook very gently, uncovered, for 1½–2 hours until you have a thick ragu, checking from time to time that it's not sticking to the bottom or drying out.

⑤ Take off the heat, stir in the chopped sage and season with salt and pepper. Allow to cool, then refrigerate in a sealed container, overnight if possible as this improves the flavour, but for at least 4 hours.

⑥ When you're ready to assemble the lasagne, preheat the oven to 190°C/Fan 170°C/Gas 5. Peel the radishes and slice them very thinly lengthways, using a mandoline if you have one, into 2mm thick slices. Put a bowl of iced water by the hob. Add the radish slices to a large pan of boiling salted water and blanch for a minute or two, then drain and refresh in the iced water. Drain again and pat dry on kitchen paper.

⑦ Spoon a layer of ragu into a shallow ovenproof dish, about 32 x 22cm and 8cm deep, and cover with a layer of white radish. Scatter over some of the mozzarella and grated Cheddar and add a few spoonfuls of crème fraîche. Repeat the ragu, radish, cheese and crème fraîche layers (you should get three of each, finishing with cheese and crème fraîche).

⑧ Stand the dish on a baking tray and place in the oven. Bake for 35–40 minutes until lightly browned on top and hot right through. Serve with a salad if you like – crunchy Romaine lettuce and tomatoes are good with this.

143

Spicy chilli with green beans

This is a real favourite in our house. It's simple to make and layered with so many deliciously spicy flavours. Green beans with cooling yoghurt and mint provide the perfect foil to the heat of the chilli. You won't even miss the rice, I promise.

Serves: 4
Carb count: 30g per person

800g best-quality minced beef
8 plum tomatoes, halved
Vegetable oil, for cooking
2 onions, diced
4 garlic cloves, grated
250g chorizo sausage (for cooking), diced
2 tbsp cumin seeds
1 tbsp chilli powder
3 tsp cracked black pepper
2 tsp ground coriander
4 celery sticks, tough strings removed, diced
400ml tin beef consommé, such as Campbell's
2–4 green chillies (depending how hot you like it), sliced, seeds and all
Juice of 1 lime
75g dark chocolate (70 per cent cocoa solids)
Sea salt and freshly ground black pepper

For the green beans:
50g butter
600g fine green beans, finely chopped
2 tbsp thick yoghurt
A handful of mint leaves (about 10g), roughly chopped

1 Preheat the oven to 190°C/Fan 170°C/Gas 5. Put the mince in a roasting tin and roast for about 40 minutes, turning every 10 minutes or so, to get a very dark, even colour all over the meat. It should be crispy and resemble instant coffee granules. You can colour the meat in a large frying pan on the hob if you prefer; just keep stirring until it is dark brown. Drain in a colander and set aside.

2 Preheat the grill to high. Place the tomatoes, cut side up, on an oven tray and grill until caramelised, about 6–8 minutes. Set aside.

3 Place a large heavy-based pan over a medium-low heat and add a good splash of oil. Add the onions and garlic and sauté, stirring from time to time, until softened, about 10–15 minutes.

4 Add the chorizo and cook until some of its fat renders and colours the onions. Stir in the cumin seeds, chilli powder, cracked black pepper and ground coriander. Cook, stirring occasionally, for 5–6 minutes.

5 Stir in the celery, browned mince and grilled tomatoes. Pour on the beef consommé and bring to the boil. Lower the heat to a simmer and cook gently, uncovered, for 1–1½ hours, until thickened to a rich chilli. Stir in the green chillies and lime juice, season with salt and remove from the heat.

To cook the beans, melt the butter in a pan over a medium-high heat. Add a good splash of water and some salt and pepper. Tip in the green beans and cook for 3–4 minutes until they are just tender. Remove from the heat and stir in the yoghurt and chopped mint.

Divide the green beans between warmed bowls, spoon on the chilli and grate some chocolate over the top to serve.

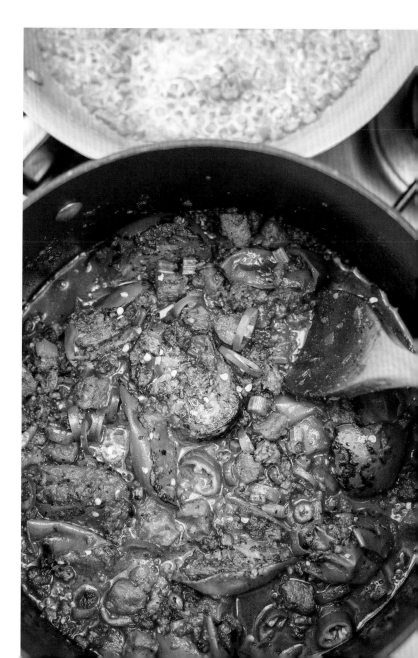

Cherry tomato stew, duck eggs and crispy beef

This is a great supper dish, but it's just as good for brunch. I like to serve a large bowl of wilted greens, such as kale or spinach, on the side.

Serves: 2

Carb count: 22g per person

Vegetable oil, for cooking
1 onion, diced
2 garlic cloves, grated
1 tbsp tomato purée
50ml red wine vinegar
1 beef stock cube
200g cherry tomatoes, halved
4 tbsp chopped pickled green chillies
2 tbsp Sriracha sauce
400g best-quality minced beef
1 tbsp cumin seeds
1 tsp garlic powder
1 tsp dried thyme
2–4 free-range duck eggs (depending how hungry you are)
Sea salt and freshly ground black pepper
Chopped parsley, to finish

1 Heat a little oil in a saucepan over a medium-low heat. Add the onion and garlic and sweat gently until soft, stirring from time to time. This should take about 10–15 minutes.

2 Stir in the tomato purée and cook for a few minutes, then add the wine vinegar and crumble in the stock cube. Turn up the heat slightly and cook for 3–4 minutes until the liquor has reduced right down.

3 Tip in the cherry tomatoes, turn the heat down a little and cook for 8–10 minutes, until the tomatoes have just broken down to form a very rough tomato sauce. Stir in the pickled chillies and Sriracha sauce, then season with salt and pepper to taste. Set aside; keep warm.

4 Heat a large, non-stick frying pan over a high heat and add a splash of oil. Fry the mince until heavily browned and crisped, stirring occasionally to break it up into crispy nuggets. When it's almost done, stir in the cumin seeds, garlic powder and thyme. Cook for 4–5 minutes and then tip the meat into a colander to drain.

5 Heat a large, non-stick frying pan over a medium-high heat, add a splash of oil and fry the eggs until the whites have set. Season.

6 Divide the tomato stew between warmed bowls and top with the duck eggs. Scatter over the crispy beef and parsley, then serve.

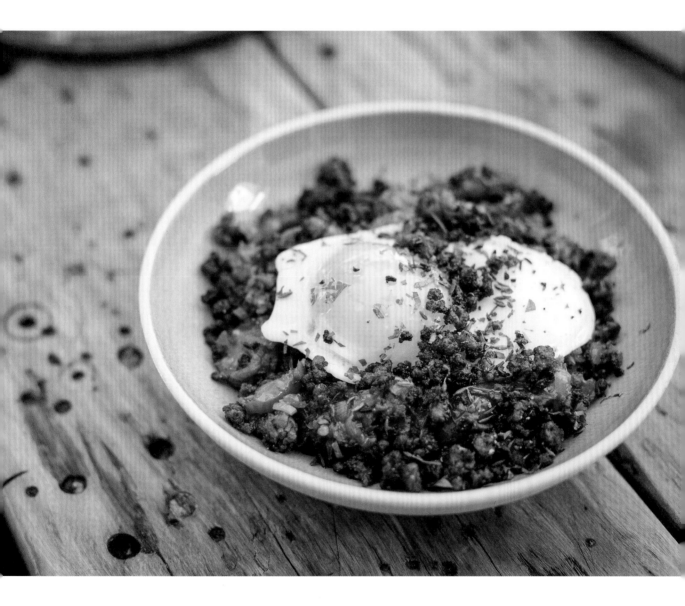

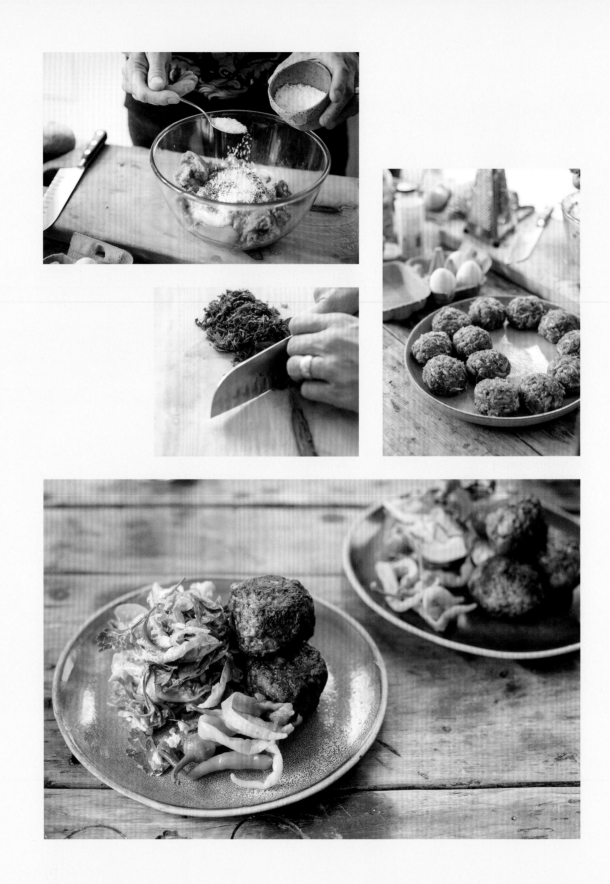

Keftedes with parsley and lemon salad

These Greek-style meatballs normally include potato or breadcrumbs, but I find peppery, low-carb turnips work very well instead and lend an excellent flavour. I like to serve the meatballs with a lively salad, which uses parsley as an ingredient in its own right.

Serves: 4

Carb count: 21g per person

For the keftedes:
350g good-quality minced beef
350g good-quality minced pork
3 large free-range eggs
3 tbsp chopped mint
2 tsp ground cinnamon
2 tsp flaky sea salt
2 tsp baking powder
1 tsp cracked black pepper
5 turnips (about 100g each), peeled
1 large onion
Olive oil, for cooking
Sea salt and freshly ground black pepper

For the salad:
2 Little Gem lettuces, leaves torn from the cores
A bunch of spring onions, trimmed and roughly chopped
A large bunch of flat-leaf parsley (about 60g), leaves picked, tough stems discarded
Finely grated zest and juice of 1 lemon
1 tbsp creamed horseradish
50ml good-quality extra virgin olive oil

To finish:
Pickled green chillies

1 Put the beef, pork, eggs, mint, cinnamon, salt, baking powder and pepper into a large bowl. Coarsely grate the turnips and onion, then squeeze in a clean tea towel to remove as much liquid as possible. Add to the bowl. Using your hands, mix until well combined. Cover and refrigerate for 30 minutes.

2 Dampen your hands a little with cold water then divide the mixture into 16 pieces and form each into a meatball.

3 Warm a generous splash of oil in a non-stick frying pan over a medium heat and fry the meatballs, turning to get a nice, even colour all over. This will take about 10–15 minutes. Remove and drain on kitchen paper.

4 While the keftedes are cooking, for the salad, mix the lettuce, spring onions, parsley leaves and lemon zest together in a bowl. Mix the creamed horseradish, lemon juice and olive oil together and season with salt and pepper. Toss the salad with this dressing.

5 Serve the keftedes as soon as they're cooked, with the salad and some pickled green chillies on the side.

Porky bolognese

This is my low-carb version of every student's favourite dish. It's one of the first things that many of us learn to cook – it's easy, it just takes a little time. If possible, make the sauce the day before you want to eat it and it'll taste even better.

Serves: 6

Carb count: 19g per person

800g good-quality minced pork
1kg ripe plum tomatoes, halved
Vegetable oil, for cooking
200g bacon lardons
2 onions, finely diced
6 garlic cloves, grated
1 tbsp cumin seeds
2 tbsp tomato purée
4 celery sticks, tough strings
     removed, diced
4 bay leaves
2 tbsp dried oregano
300g button mushrooms, stalks
     removed, caps halved
500ml beef or chicken stock
200ml red wine
A small bunch of sage, tough
     stems discarded, leaves
     roughly chopped
Sea salt and freshly ground
     black pepper

For the spaghetti:
4–6 courgettes (about 700–800g
     in total)
75g butter

To serve:
Freshly grated Parmesan cheese

1 Preheat the oven to 200°C/Fan 180°C/Gas 6. Season the minced pork well with salt and pepper. Place in a roasting tin and cook in the oven for 25–30 minutes until very crisp and heavily browned, stirring every 10 minutes or so to ensure it colours evenly.

2 Put the tomatoes, cut side up, in another roasting tin and roast alongside the pork for 25 minutes, until they start to colour and shrivel around the edges. Remove from the oven and set aside.

3 Warm a little oil in a large saucepan over a medium-low heat. Add the lardons, onions and garlic and sweat gently, stirring from time to time, for 10–15 minutes until the onions are soft. Add the cumin seeds and cook, stirring, for a couple of minutes, then stir in the tomato purée and cook for a further 3–4 minutes. Add the celery, bay leaves and oregano. Cook, stirring, for 1–2 minutes.

4 Add the minced pork, roasted tomatoes and mushrooms to the pan. Stir, then pour in the stock and wine. Bring to the boil, lower the heat and add some salt and pepper. Simmer very gently, uncovered, for 1–2 hours, until thickened to a rich ragu, stirring from time to time to make sure it doesn't stick. Remove from the heat and stir in the chopped sage. Taste to check the seasoning.

⑤ When ready to eat, reheat the pork ragu. Meanwhile, pass the courgettes through a spiralizer to make thin 'spaghetti'. In a large saucepan, warm 75ml water with the butter and a little salt and pepper. Add the courgette spaghetti and heat gently until just warmed through; don't overcook them.

⑥ Drain the courgette spaghetti well and divide between warmed bowls. Spoon on the porky bolognese and scatter over some grated Parmesan to serve.

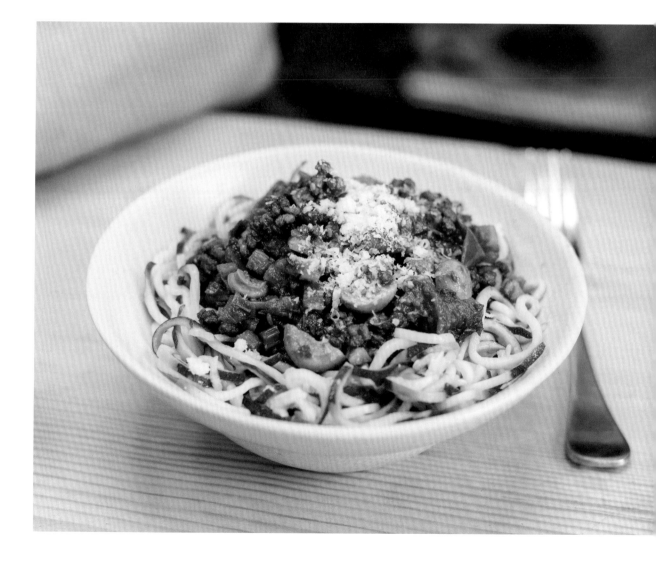

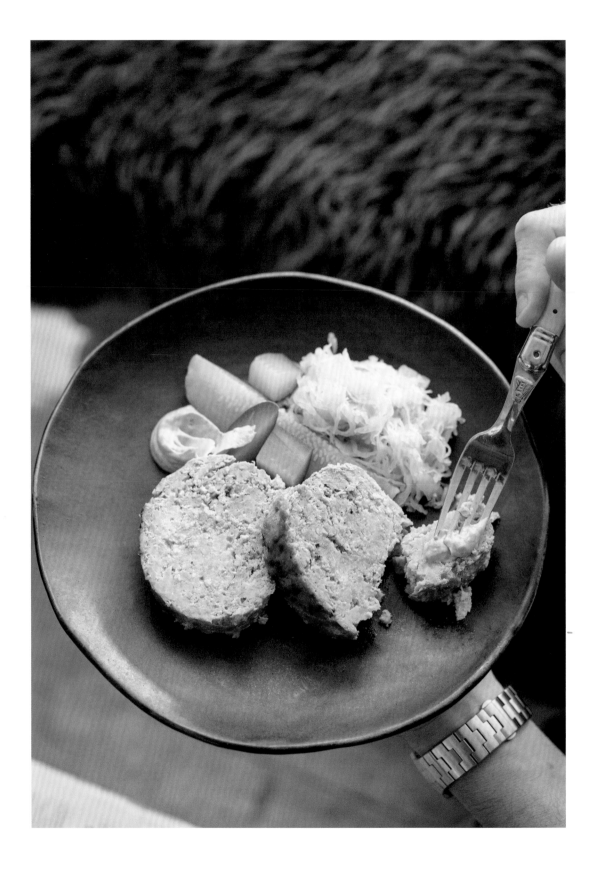

Garlic sausage meatloaf

The gutsy flavours and textures of a classic Polish sausage inspired this recipe, but I wanted the ease of baking the mix in a loaf tin rather than the faff of stuffing sausage skins. The result is pretty good I think, and straightforward – especially if you get your butcher to mince the meat for you. Serve it hot or cold, with your favourite condiments and a salad. I also like a bowl of sauerkraut on the side.

Serves: 4–6

Carb count: 7–5g per person

800g minced pork shoulder
100g minced pork back fat
250g minced raw gammon
1 garlic bulb (about 8–12 cloves),
    peeled and grated
2 tsp salt
1 tsp cracked black pepper
¼–½ nutmeg, finely grated
2 tbsp creamed horseradish
2 tbsp Sriracha sauce
1 tsp Worcestershire sauce
1 tsp Tabasco sauce

To serve:
American-style or German mustard
Tomato ketchup
Dill pickles
Sauerkraut or salad

1 Put the pork shoulder, back fat, gammon, garlic, salt, pepper and nutmeg into a large bowl and work the mixture together using your hands to combine, until it tightens and firms up.

2 Pack the meat mixture into a non-stick (or parchment-lined) 1kg loaf tin. Cover with foil and leave to rest for 10 minutes.

3 Preheat the oven to 180°C/Fan 160°C/Gas 4. Stand the loaf tin on an oven tray and bake for 40–45 minutes. Remove from the oven and lift off the foil.

4 In a clean bowl, mix together the creamed horseradish, Sriracha, Worcestershire and Tabasco sauces with a splash of water.

5 Preheat the grill to medium-high. Brush the horseradish glaze over the top of the meatloaf. Place under the grill for 5–10 minutes, until the top has turned a lovely, golden brown colour. Set aside to rest for 10 minutes.

6 Carefully remove the meatloaf from the tin. Serve it in thick slices with your favourite condiments and some sauerkraut or a salad on the side.

Pork kebabs and spicy cauliflower couscous

This is my play on that favourite post-pub, late-night classic, the kebab. It has the wonderful, bold, strong, delicious flavours of Greek food that I enjoy so much, and on a summer's day it works brilliantly on the barbecue.

Serves: 2

Carb count: 26g per person

For the kebabs:
500g good-quality minced pork
1 red onion, diced
3 garlic cloves, grated
3 tbsp fennel seeds, toasted in a dry frying pan until fragrant then lightly crushed with a pestle and mortar
Finely grated zest of 1 orange
2 tsp salt
Vegetable oil, for cooking

For the cauliflower couscous:
1 cauliflower (about 600g), broken into florets
1 tsp ground cumin
1 tsp cracked black pepper
½ tsp chilli powder
2 tbsp extra virgin olive oil
A bunch of coriander (about 25g), finely chopped, tender stems and all
Sea salt and freshly ground black pepper

For the seasoned yoghurt:
3 tbsp thick Greek yoghurt
1 tbsp tahini
Juice of ½ lemon
1 tbsp extra virgin olive oil

1 Put the pork, red onion, garlic, fennel seeds, orange zest and salt into a bowl. Mix with your hands until well combined and slightly firmed up.

2 Shape into 10 small, sausage-shaped kebabs – or fewer, larger ones if you like. Place on a plate, cover with cling film, and refrigerate for at least an hour or overnight, to allow them to firm up and to let the flavours develop.

3 Preheat the oven to 200°C/Fan 180°C/Gas 6. Put the cauliflower into a food processor and blitz until it resembles couscous. Mix in the cumin, cracked black pepper and chilli powder. Spread out on a baking tray and trickle over the olive oil. Cook in the oven for 15–20 minutes until dried out, giving it a stir halfway through. Leave the cauliflower couscous to cool on the baking tray.

4 Tip the cooled couscous into a bowl, season with salt and pepper and stir in the coriander.

5 In a separate bowl, mix together the yoghurt, tahini, lemon juice and olive oil. Season with salt and pepper to taste.

6 Heat a large, non-stick frying pan over a medium-high heat, add a splash of oil, and fry the pork kebabs for 3–4 minutes on each side. Serve with the spicy cauliflower couscous and seasoned yoghurt.

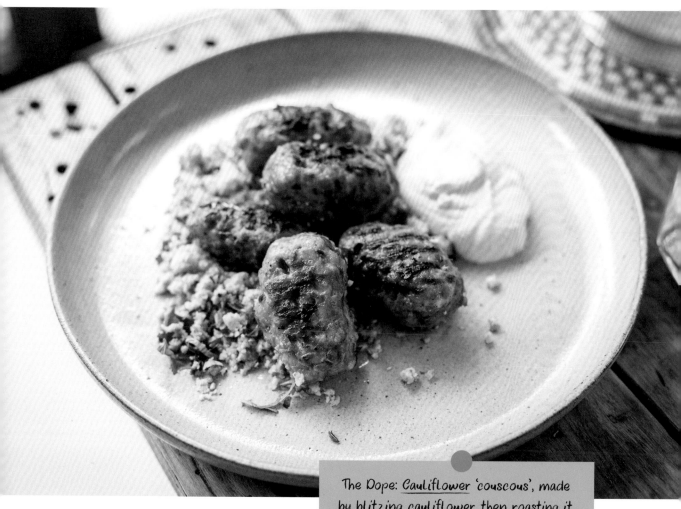

The Dope: <u>Cauliflower</u> 'couscous', made by blitzing cauliflower then roasting it and pepping it up with spices and herbs, is a great low-carb alternative to rice, pasta or couscous.

Crispy vinegar pork with cauliflower purée

Rich, silky smooth cauliflower makes a sophisticated contrast to tasty little nuggets of crispy minced pork, cool mint and toasted sesame seeds. This great little dish also works well as a starter, in smaller portions.

Serves: 4

Carb count: 16g per person

For the vinegar pork:
800g good-quality minced pork
Vegetable oil, for cooking
1 onion, finely diced
2 tbsp cumin seeds
3 garlic cloves, grated
1 tsp cracked black pepper
100ml sherry vinegar
250ml chicken stock
Finely grated zest of 1 lemon
½ bunch of mint (about 10g),
    tough stems removed, leaves
    shredded
Sea salt and freshly ground
    black pepper

For the cauliflower purée:
1 cauliflower (about 600g
    prepared weight), cut into florets
40g butter
1 onion, diced
4 garlic cloves, grated
150ml double cream
100g tahini
Cayenne pepper

To finish:
1 tbsp sesame seeds, toasted
    until golden in a dry frying pan
A handful of mint leaves

1 Preheat the oven to 200°C/Fan 180°C/Gas 6. Season the minced pork well with salt and pepper. Place in a roasting tin and cook in the oven for about 25–30 minutes until very crisp and heavily browned, stirring every 10 minutes or so to ensure it colours evenly. You can also brown the meat in a large frying pan over a medium-high heat on the hob if you prefer; just keep stirring until it is well browned. Tip the mince into a colander and set aside to drain.

2 For the cauliflower purée, bring a large pan of salted water to the boil and blanch the florets until just soft, about 4–5 minutes. Drain and pat dry with a clean tea towel or kitchen paper.

3 Melt the butter in a large frying pan or saucepan over a medium-low heat. Add the onion and garlic and sweat gently, stirring from time to time, for 10–15 minutes until softened. Add the blanched cauliflower and stir. Pour in the cream and bring to the boil. Lower the heat and cook for 2–3 minutes.

4 Tip the cauliflower into a food processor. Add the tahini, season well with salt and cayenne pepper and blitz until very smooth. If there's time, pass it through a fine sieve too, to give it an extra silky texture. Set aside.

To finish the pork, place a frying pan over a medium-high heat. Drizzle in a little oil and add the onion. Cook for 10–15 minutes, stirring from time to time, until golden brown. Add the cumin seeds, garlic and cracked black pepper. Cook, stirring, for 2–3 minutes and then add the browned mince.

Pour on the sherry vinegar, bring to the boil and reduce down to a glaze. Pour in the stock, bring to the boil again and let bubble until the crispy pork is glazed and sticky. Add the lemon zest and shredded mint and stir through.

Serve the crispy pork with the cauliflower purée on the side. Finish with a scattering of sesame seeds and mint leaves.

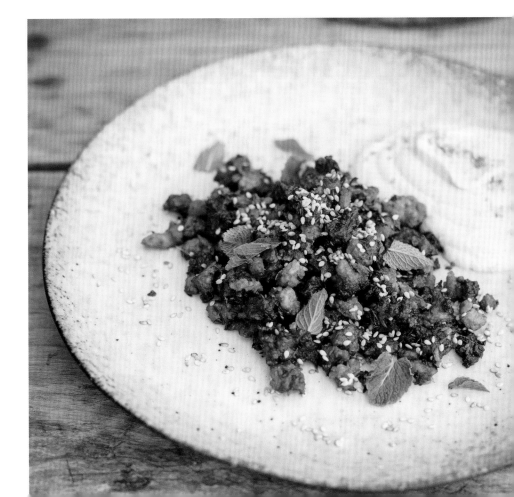

Toulouse sausage loaf with fried pickle salad

This garlicky, slightly spicy sausage loaf is delicious both hot and cold, so enjoy it for supper one day and keep some leftovers for a quick lunch the next. Frying the dill pickles adds an unexpected but really tasty dimension to the salad.

Serves: 6
Carb count: 20g per person

For the sausage loaf:
750g minced pork shoulder
250g minced pork belly
100g dried onion flakes
5 garlic cloves, grated
3 tbsp chopped parsley
2 tbsp cracked black pepper
1 tbsp salt
1 tbsp fennel seeds
1 tbsp dried oregano
1 tsp cayenne pepper
A little vegetable oil, for cooking and oiling

For the fried pickle salad:
A jar of large dill pickles (about 650g)
Vegetable oil, for frying
8–10 marinated artichokes in olive oil
10 large pickled green chillies
A bunch of dill (about 20g), chopped
1 tbsp medium-hot German mustard

1 To make the sausage loaf, put all of the meat and flavouring ingredients into a large bowl and work together with your hands, until well combined and firmed up slightly. To check the seasoning, break off a small piece and fry it in a little oil in a small pan until cooked through. Taste and then adjust the seasoning of the main mixture if necessary.

2 Oil a large piece of foil and place the sausage mixture in the middle. Form into a tightly packed sausage, about 25cm long. Wrap very tightly in the foil and secure the ends. Place on a baking tray and rest in the fridge for at least 2 hours.

3 Preheat the oven to 180°C/Fan 160°C/Gas 4. Bake the sausage loaf for 40 minutes, then take out of the oven and carefully remove the foil. Return the unwrapped sausage loaf to the oven and cook for a further 15 minutes until it is a rich, golden brown. Leave to rest for 10 minutes.

4 Meanwhile, prepare the fried pickles. Halve the dill pickles lengthways and pat dry on kitchen paper. Heat up a non-stick frying pan over a medium-high heat and add a little oil. Fry the dill pickles, seed side down, until toasty and golden brown. You may need to do this in batches. Transfer the pickles to a bowl; keep warm.

Add the artichokes to the frying pan and gently warm through, then return the fried pickles to the pan and add the chillies, chopped dill and mustard. Stir to mix.

6 Cut the sausage loaf into thick slices and serve with the fried pickle salad.

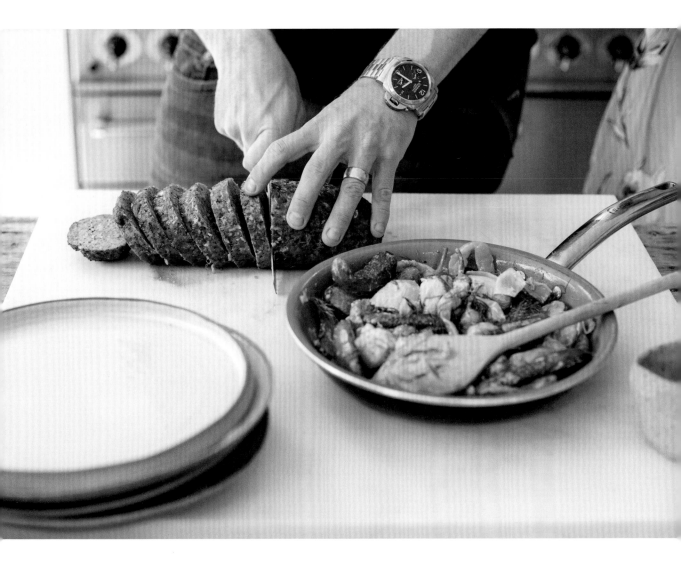

Rich and comforting

BRAISES
&
STEWS

SLOW COOKING IS FASCINATING. To me, the way raw meat is transformed into a rich, silky, intensely flavoured dinner is quite magical. With time and gentle heat, you can turn the most humble cuts of meat into something very special.

In everything I do, I seek to add deep, rich flavours. Infusing stocks and sauces with herbs, spices and seasonings is just the start. The lower and slower you cook the dish, the more opportunity those flavours have to permeate the meat with their aromas. When you cook something over many hours, it transforms into something so unctuous and tender, it absolutely doesn't feel like diet food. Not the old-school kind of diet food which would leave you feeling miserable and deprived, anyway.

These dishes are special – the sort of beautiful, well-cooked food that makes you feel nurtured and loved. The only difference from familiar comfort food is that you're not serving them with a heap of mash or chips on the side.

When I was devising my regime and choosing the recipes for this book, one thought was very important to me: few of us eat alone. We eat with our families, our mates, our colleagues at work, and if you're the one on the diet, you don't want to feel like the weirdo at the end of the table diving into a carton of carrots and hummus.

I knew that for me, and for others like me, to succeed in this new approach to eating, all of the dishes had to work for everyone. I had to be able to sit down with my wife Beth, and with friends at the weekend, and tuck into exactly the same thing as they were eating, with none of us feeling compromised. One of the things I'm proudest of is that if you serve up any of the dishes in this book no one will know it's 'diet food'. This is because it is not – it's just really good food that happens to be low-carb.

Don't be put off by some of the lengthy cooking times in this chapter – the oven is doing most of the work. While the cooking time for the braised beef with horseradish (page 183), lamb shank hot pot (page 174) and pork stew with a smoked cheese crust (page 191) may be around 4 hours, the hands-on time is only about 20 minutes. The great flavour comes from the slow, low cooking and not from any elaborate prep, so once you've put it all together you can bung it in the oven and just get on with your life until dinner.

And for those days when you just don't have the time, there are some lovely, satisfying recipes such as beef stroganoff (page 178) which taste slow-cooked and tender, but are actually fairly quick to make, start to finish.

Don't overlook the large chunks of meat, such as the spiced lamb shoulder on page 176, if you're cooking for only a small number of people. For my low-carb regime, delicious, meaty leftovers are your friends. They're great just with a few salad leaves and maybe some pickles for a quick lunch, or you can combine them with other recipes in this book. For example, try flaking leftover slow-cooked lamb and combining it with the spicy Indian egg rolls (page 99) for a packed lunch that will be the envy of your office. That's what I call winning.

<u>Dopamine and meat</u>

Meat proteins are high in the amino acids which promote dopamine production in the brain. Choose well-reared, free-range animals whenever you can. A little meat can go a long way, so focus on quality rather than quantity. A smaller portion of something really wonderful can be deeply satisfying.

Poached salmon, samphire and seaweed

Sometimes you want a dish that's both light and fragrant but gives you something substantial too, and this simple salmon stew definitely fits the bill. Not only is it deeply satisfying, it looks beautiful too.

Serves: 2

Carb count: 16g per person

20g dried seaweed, such as
    wakame
Vegetable oil, for cooking
4 garlic cloves, sliced
1 tsp freshly grated ginger
2 tbsp freshly grated horseradish
50ml rice wine vinegar
100g shiitake mushrooms, sliced
1–2 turnips (200g total weight),
    peeled and very thinly sliced,
    ideally with a mandoline
½ tsp ground white pepper
75g samphire
2 salmon fillets (about 200g each),
    skinned and pin-boned
1–2 tbsp toasted sesame oil

1 Put the seaweed into a bowl and pour on 1 litre warm water (from a pre-boiled kettle). Leave to rehydrate for 20 minutes. Drain the seaweed in a sieve set over a bowl then tip onto a plate; reserve the soaking liquid.

2 Warm a saucepan over a medium heat and add a splash of oil. Toss in the garlic and toast until it just starts to turn golden brown – don't take it too far, you don't want to scorch it. Add the ginger and horseradish and stir for a few seconds. Pour in the rice wine vinegar and bring to the boil. Add the reserved seaweed liquid and bring to a simmer.

3 Tip in the shiitake mushrooms and poach for 2–3 minutes. Add the sliced turnips and cook for a further 4–5 minutes. Stir in the white pepper then add the seaweed and samphire.

4 Place the salmon fillets in the hot broth, cover the pan and immediately take it off the heat. Leave the salmon to poach in the residual heat for 5–6 minutes.

5 Serve immediately in warmed bowls, with a little toasted sesame oil trickled over the top.

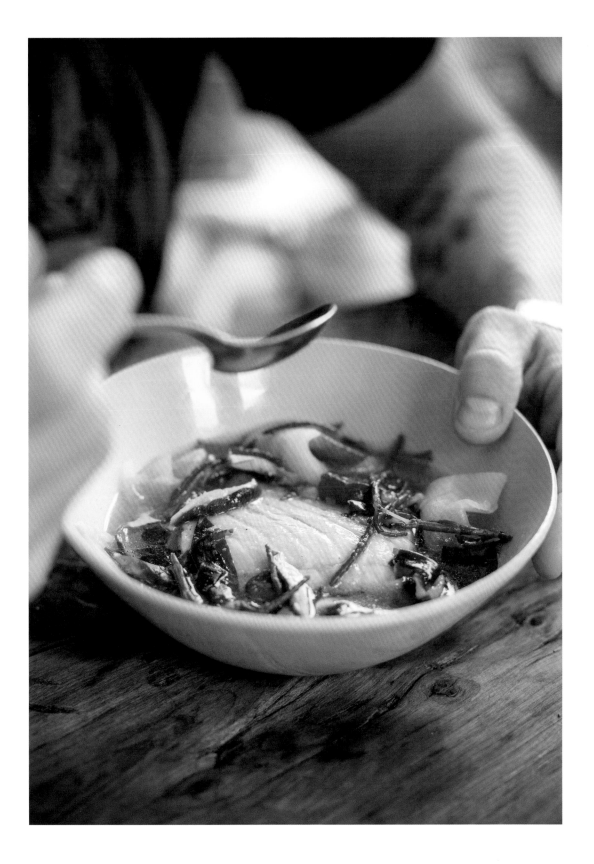

Moroccan chicken with cauliflower couscous

Whenever I'm missing high-carb rice, I turn to cauliflower 'couscous' – it's very tasty, easy to make and goes brilliantly with all sorts of main courses. Here, I pair it with chicken, which I fry really hard initially, to give it that moreish crispness. This dish is good warm or cold, so it's ideal for a substantial packed lunch the next day too.

Serves: 4

Carb count: 28g per person

4 tbsp olive oil
8 large free-range chicken thighs, skinned and de-boned
2 onions, diced
4 garlic cloves, grated
4cm knob of fresh ginger, grated
2 tsp ras el hanout
2 tsp salt
1 tsp cracked black pepper
1 tsp ground cinnamon
½ tsp ground turmeric
400ml chicken stock
1 preserved lemon, chopped
1 tbsp clear honey

For the cauliflower couscous:
1 cauliflower (about 600g)
½ bunch of flat-leaf parsley (about 15g)
½ bunch of mint (about 15g)
½ bunch of coriander (about 15g)
150g blanched hazelnuts, toasted until golden and roughly crushed
2 tomatoes, cored, deseeded and diced
1 red onion, very finely diced
4 tbsp good-quality extra virgin olive oil
Finely grated zest of 1 lemon
Sea salt and freshly ground black pepper

To serve:
Thick yoghurt

1 Heat the olive oil in a large, heavy-bottomed sauté pan or flameproof casserole over a medium heat. Fry the chicken thighs in batches, flat side down, for 15 minutes until browned and crisped underneath. Remove from the pan; set aside.

2 Reduce the heat and add the onions, garlic and ginger to the pan. Stir to mix in any crisp bits from the chicken and sauté gently until softened, about 10–15 minutes. Stir in the ras el hanout, salt, cracked pepper, cinnamon and turmeric.

3 Return the chicken to the pan. Stir in the stock, preserved lemon and honey. Increase the heat a little and bring to a simmer. Cook until the stock has reduced right down and the chicken is nicely glazed. Remove from the heat; set aside.

4 While the chicken is cooking, preheat the oven to 200°C/Fan 180°C/Gas 6. For the couscous, break the cauliflower into florets and blitz in a food processor until it resembles couscous. Spread out on a baking tray and roast to dry out for 15–20 minutes, giving it a stir halfway through. Leave to cool on the tray.

5 Discard any tough stems from the parsley, mint and coriander and then roughly chop the herbs. Tip into a large bowl.

6 Add the cauliflower couscous to the herbs, along with all the remaining ingredients, seasoning with salt and pepper to taste. Toss well to combine. Serve the chicken with the cauliflower couscous and thick yoghurt.

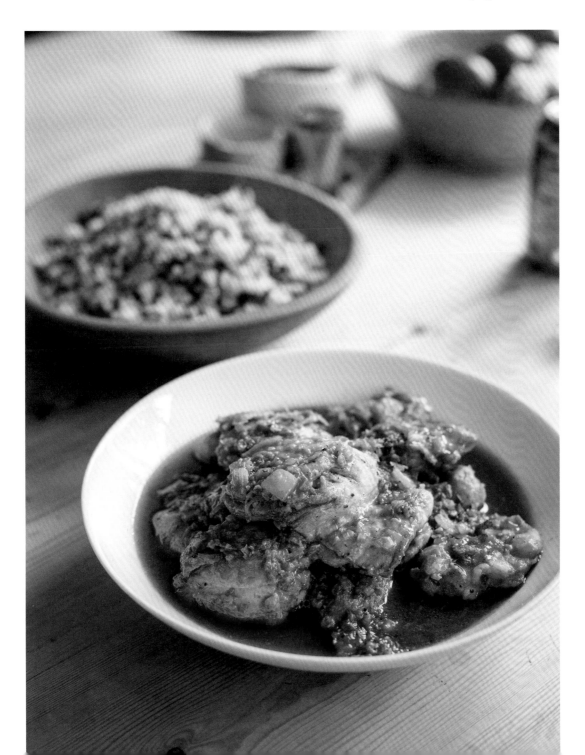

Cider-poached chicken with apple slaw

This is a wonderfully simple dish. With relatively few flavouring ingredients, it's really worth seeking out the very best chicken you can find – it will make all the difference to the end result. Before you get started, you'll also need to make sure you have a heavy-bottomed casserole or pan with a lid that is large enough to take the whole chicken.

Serves: 4

Carb count: 31g per person

For the poached chicken:
1 organic or free-range chicken (about 1.4kg)
500ml dry cider
A bunch of thyme (6–8 sprigs), tied with kitchen string
1 medium Savoy cabbage, cut into quarters, trimmed with core intact
200g bacon lardons
2 tbsp mustard seeds, toasted in a dry frying pan just until they start to pop
200ml chicken gravy (I make it with Bisto chicken gravy granules)
2 tbsp Dijon mustard
2 tbsp chopped sage leaves
Sea salt and freshly ground black pepper

For the apple slaw:
1 small onion, halved and very thinly sliced
1 kohlrabi, peeled and cut into julienne
1 tsp flaky sea salt
3 Granny Smith apples (unpeeled)
1 red apple, peeled
Finely grated zest of 1 lemon
3 tbsp thick mayonnaise

① Preheat the oven to 170°C/Fan 150°C/Gas 3. Place the chicken in a heavy-bottomed ovenproof pan or flameproof casserole then pour on the cider. Add the thyme and some salt and pepper. Bring the cider to the boil, put the lid on and place in the oven. Cook for 1½ hours.

② Meanwhile, make the apple slaw. Toss the onion and kohlrabi with the flaky salt to mix well and leave to stand for 10 minutes. Rinse under cold running water, then pat dry with a clean tea towel or kitchen paper and place in a bowl.

③ Using the coarse side of a box grater, grate all 4 apples onto a clean tea towel. Wrap the grated apples in the tea towel and squeeze out their juice over a bowl; reserve the juice. Add the grated apples and lemon zest to the kohlrabi and onion and toss to mix. Add the mayonnaise and combine well. Cover and refrigerate until needed.

④ After 1½ hours, take the pan or casserole from the oven. Carefully lift out the chicken and place in a warmed roasting tin. Cover with foil and leave to rest in a warm place. Discard the thyme from the poaching liquor.

5 Place the pan back on a medium heat and bring to the boil. Pour in the reserved apple juice and let bubble to reduce by two-thirds. Add the cabbage, lardons and mustard seeds. Put the lid back on, lower the heat and cook gently for 8–10 minutes, until the cabbage and bacon are just cooked. Stir in the gravy, mustard and sage and bring to a simmer.

6 Remove the foil from the chicken. If you have a cook's blowtorch, use it to colour the skin deep golden brown all over.

7 Joint the chicken and serve on warmed plates with the poached cabbage and bacon spooned around it and the apple slaw on the side.

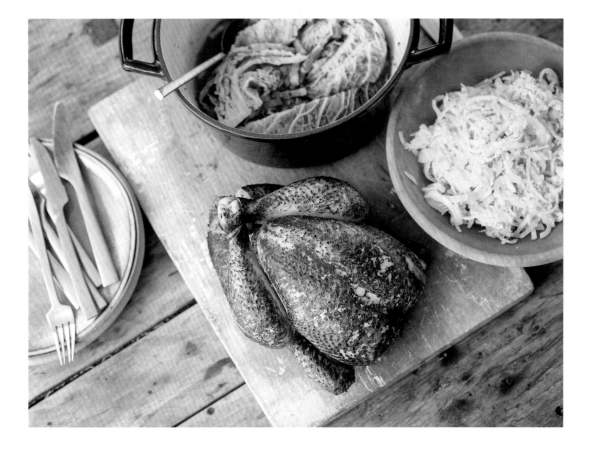

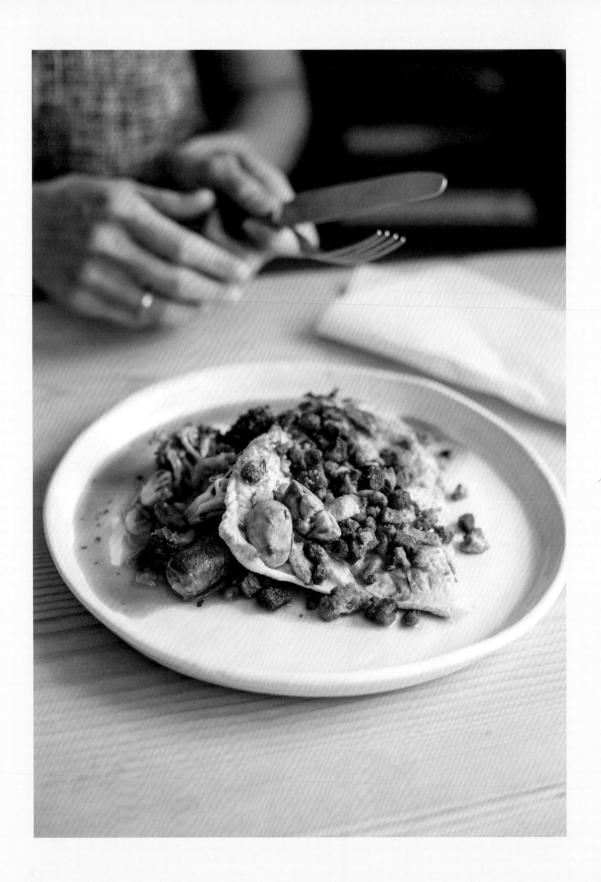

Turkey stew with wasabi pork crunch

This is such a brilliant supper. If you grab a couple of turkey escalopes from the meat counter on your way home from work, you can knock up this quick and easy dish in next to no time. Turkey is an under-used meat too, so it's nice to give it an outing.

Serves: 2

Carb count: 34g per person

Vegetable oil, for cooking
2 turkey breast fillets (about 200g each)
2 onions, halved and sliced
2 garlic cloves, grated
½ tbsp dried sage
½ head of broccoli (about 180g), cut into small florets
100g cooked cocktail sausages
A bunch of chives (about 20g), chopped
A bunch of sage (about 15g), stems discarded, leaves chopped
100g pancetta, diced quite small
70g pork scratchings, broken up a little
2 tbsp wasabi powder
1 tsp thyme leaves
250ml chicken gravy (I make it with Bisto chicken gravy granules)
100ml white wine
100g button mushrooms, stalks removed, caps halved
Sea salt and freshly ground black pepper

1 Heat a non-stick frying pan over a medium-high heat and drizzle in a little oil. Season the turkey fillets with salt and pepper and place in the pan. Cook until lightly browned on both sides, about 3–4 minutes per side. Remove and set aside.

2 Heat a little more oil in the pan and add the onions, garlic and dried sage. Sauté gently for about 10–15 minutes until the onions are softened, stirring from time to time.

3 Preheat the oven to 190°C/Fan 170°C/Gas 5. Tip the onions into a shallow ovenproof dish, about 25cm square. Stir in the broccoli florets, cocktail sausages, chives and chopped sage.

4 Fry the diced pancetta in a dry frying pan over a medium heat until crisp, then drain on kitchen paper. Tip into a bowl and add the pork scratchings, wasabi powder and thyme leaves. Mix together.

5 Lay the turkey fillets on top of the onions, broccoli and cocktail sausages. Mix the chicken gravy with the wine and pour over the turkey. Scatter the pork crunch over the top. Bake in the oven for 20–25 minutes, until the broccoli is cooked and the topping is nice and crunchy. Serve immediately.

Fragrant steamed duck with cantaloupe salad

I love this hot salad so much. It has such a great balance of sweet, spice and salt, and the texture of the cold melon combines wonderfully with the hot, silky, slow-cooked duck. Gorgeous!

Serves: 2–4
Carb count: 23–11g per person

For the duck:
1 oven-ready duck (about 2kg)
4 star anise
1 tsp Szechuan peppercorns
1 tsp coriander seeds
1 tbsp flaky sea salt
1 tsp Chinese five-spice powder
1 tsp ground ginger
2 tbsp vegetable oil

For the salad:
1 cantaloupe melon
1 Chinese leaf lettuce, shredded
A bunch of spring onions, trimmed
   and finely sliced
A bunch of coriander (about 25g),
   leaves picked from stems
A bunch of mint (about 30g), tough
   stems discarded, leaves torn
2 tbsp sesame seeds, toasted in
   a dry frying pan until lightly
   golden
2 red chillies, sliced, seeds and all
Finely grated zest and juice of
   2 limes
2 tbsp Thai fish sauce
2 tbsp dark soy sauce
2 tsp sesame oil

① Preheat the oven to 150°C/Fan 130°C/Gas 2. Score the duck skin all over.

② In a dry frying pan over a medium heat, toast the star anise, Szechuan peppercorns, coriander seeds and flaky sea salt until lightly browned, about 2–3 minutes. Cool and then crush using a pestle and mortar. Add the Chinese five-spice powder and ground ginger and mix well.

③ Rub the spice mix into the duck skin then stand the duck on a rack in a deep-sided roasting tin. Pour 500ml water into the bottom of the tin. Cover the whole tin with foil and seal tightly around the rim. Place in the oven to steam-roast for 5 hours. Remove from the oven and set aside to rest for about 20 minutes.

④ Meanwhile, for the salad, peel, halve and deseed the melon, then cut into large chunks. Place in a bowl with the Chinese leaf, spring onions, coriander, mint, sesame seeds, red chillies and lime zest. Toss gently to mix.

⑤ For the dressing, mix the lime juice, fish sauce, soy sauce and sesame oil together in a small bowl. Trickle the dressing over the salad and toss to combine.

Lift off the foil and brush the duck with the oil. If you have a cook's blowtorch, use it to brown the skin all over and crisp it slightly. Flake the duck and serve immediately with the salad.

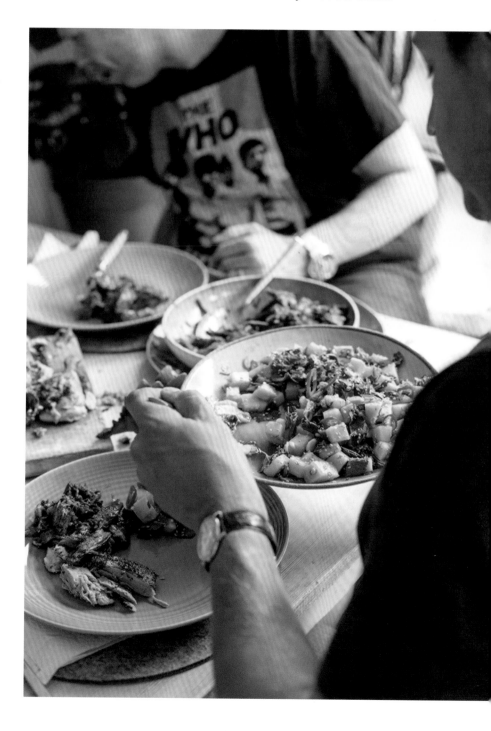

Lamb shank hot pot

Here I've recreated that old-school favourite, Lancashire hot pot, using a different cut of lamb. Shanks provide you with perfect portion control – one each. Crammed with vegetables too, this one-pot dinner is a real crowd pleaser.

Serves: 4
Carb count: 17g per person

Vegetable oil, for cooking
4 lamb shanks (about 200g each),
    French trimmed (get your
    butcher to do this for you)
6 small onions, halved
1 garlic bulb (about 8–12 cloves),
    peeled and sliced
1 large swede, peeled and diced
150g crumbled goat's cheese
1 tbsp cracked black pepper
2 tsp thyme leaves
500ml lamb stock
4 large turnips (about 200g each),
    peeled and thinly sliced
50g butter, diced
Sea salt and freshly ground
    black pepper

 Heat a good splash of oil in a large flameproof casserole over a medium-high heat. Season the lamb shanks with a little salt then fry them two at a time until deeply and evenly coloured. Don't hurry the process – searing the meat properly helps to create that deep, delicious flavour. Drain off the rendered fat. Set the lamb shanks aside.

Turn the heat down a bit and add a splash more oil to the casserole, followed by the onions, garlic and a pinch of salt. Cook gently for about 10–12 minutes until golden and softened. Remove from the heat and return the lamb shanks to the pan, placing them on top of the onions with the bones pointing upwards.

Preheat the oven to 150°C/Fan 130°C/Gas 2. In a bowl, combine the swede, goat's cheese, pepper and thyme, then pack it around the lamb shanks. Pour in the stock. Fan the turnip slices in a circle over the swede and around the lamb shanks then dot with the butter.

Put the lid on or, if that's not possible because the shank bones are poking up too high, cover with foil and seal tightly. Cook in the oven for 1½ hours, then remove the lid or foil and return to the oven for a further 1½ hours until the lamb is soft, covering with foil if it browns too quickly. The turnips will be crispy on the top.

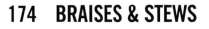

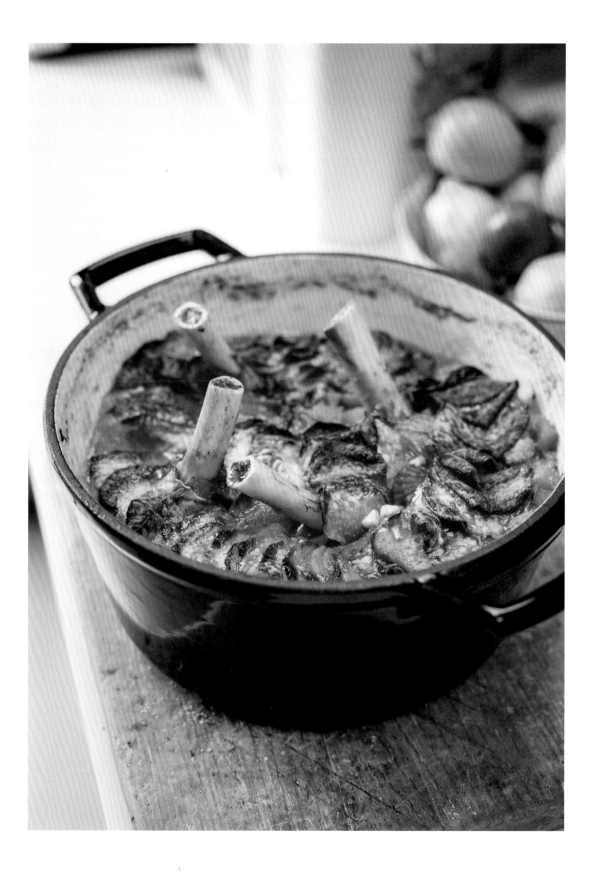

Spiced lamb shoulder with curried cauliflower

For me, slow-cooked spiced shoulder of lamb is one of the all-time great comfort foods, and if you make the spice paste yourself it's always a winner.

Serves: 4

Carb count: 19g per person

For the lamb:
10 dried red chillies
6 garlic cloves, peeled
2 tbsp red wine vinegar
2 tsp ground coriander
2 tsp ground cumin
2 tsp smoked paprika
2 tsp curry powder
2 tsp sea salt
70ml olive oil
1 shoulder of lamb (about 2kg), bone in

For the curried cauliflower:
Vegetable oil, for cooking
1 large cauliflower (about 800g), cut into florets
250g paneer or halloumi, cut into 2cm cubes
1 onion, halved and thinly sliced
4cm knob of fresh ginger, grated
2 garlic cloves, grated
2 tsp curry powder
2 tsp ground turmeric
500g broad-leaf spinach, tough stalks removed
Sea salt and freshly ground black pepper

To serve (optional):
Thick yoghurt

1 Put the dried chillies into a bowl, cover with boiling water and leave to rehydrate and cool. Drain the chillies, reserving the soaking water.

2 Put the chillies into a food processor with the garlic, wine vinegar, spices, salt and olive oil. Blend to a paste, adding a little of the chilli soaking water if it is too thick.

3 Score 1cm deep cuts all over the lamb joint. Massage the spice paste all over the lamb then wrap it tightly in cling film and place on a tray. Leave to marinate in the fridge for 8 hours.

4 Preheat the oven to 140°C/Fan 120°C/Gas 1. Unwrap the lamb and place in a roasting tin. Cook for 4–4½ hours until the meat is so tender you can easily flake it from the bone with a fork. Set aside to rest for 30 minutes.

5 Meanwhile, heat a good splash of oil in a large, heavy pan over a medium-high heat. Add the cauliflower and cook for 15–20 minutes until golden brown all over, stirring as little as possible. Tip onto kitchen paper to drain.

6 Add another splash of oil to the pan and fry the cheese over a medium heat until browned all over. Remove and drain on kitchen paper.

7 Drizzle a little more oil into the pan and add the onion, ginger and garlic. Sauté gently over a medium-low heat for about 10–15 minutes, until softened. Add the curry powder and turmeric and cook, stirring, for a minute.

Return the cauliflower to the pan and pour in 200ml water. Simmer for a couple of minutes, then add the cheese, followed by the spinach and cook briefly, stirring, until the spinach has just wilted. Season with salt to taste.

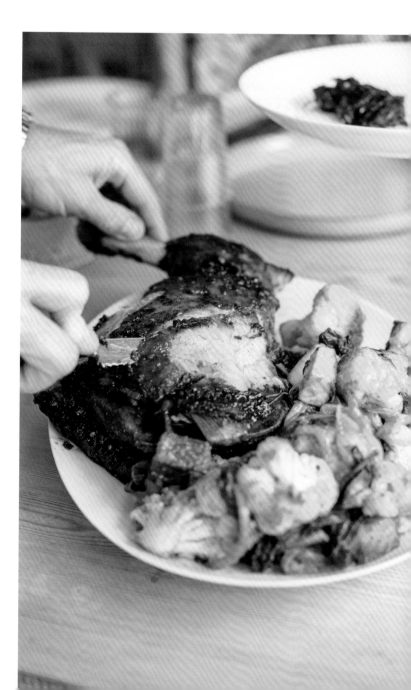 Serve the lamb with the curried cauliflower, and thick yoghurt on the side if you like.

Beef stroganoff

This recipe is so rich and luxurious it feels special, and yet it's easy to make. Beef fillet tails are a great cut – tender and full of flavour – but feel free to swap them for sirloin, rump or rib eye steak if you prefer.

Serves: 2
Carb count: 23g per person

Vegetable oil, for cooking
2 beef fillet tails (about 200g each)
50g butter
1 onion, sliced
3 garlic cloves, grated
2 tsp smoked paprika
1 beef stock cube
1 tbsp tomato purée
400ml tin beef consommé, such
    as Campbell's
1 tbsp Dijon mustard
150g chestnut mushrooms, stalks
    removed, caps quartered
3 tbsp crème fraîche
75g gherkins, chopped
Juice of ½ lemon
60g packet of pork scratchings,
    roughly crushed
4 tbsp chopped chervil
2 tbsp dried onion flakes
Sea salt and freshly ground
    black pepper

1 Heat a large, heavy-bottomed sauté pan or frying pan over a medium-high heat and add a little oil. Season the beef fillets with salt and pepper and place in the pan. Sear well all over until dark brown in colour. Add the butter and baste the steaks until cooked to medium-rare, about 2–3 minutes each side. Remove from the pan and leave to rest on a plate.

2 Lower the heat under the pan to medium-low, add the onion and garlic and sweat gently for 10–15 minutes until softened, stirring from time to time. Add the smoked paprika, crumble in the stock cube and cook, stirring, for 2–3 minutes. Stir in the tomato purée and cook for 1–2 minutes.

3 Pour in the beef consommé and stir in the mustard. Turn the heat up to medium-high, bring to the boil and add the mushrooms. Cook until the sauce is reduced to a rich glaze, then lower the heat and stir in the crème fraîche. Season with salt and pepper.

4 Cut the beef into thick strips and return to the pan, with any juices from the plate. Stir in the gherkins and lemon juice. Take off the heat.

5 Mix the crushed pork scratchings with the chopped chervil and onion flakes. Spoon the stroganoff into warmed bowls, sprinkle over the pork crunch mixture and serve straight away.

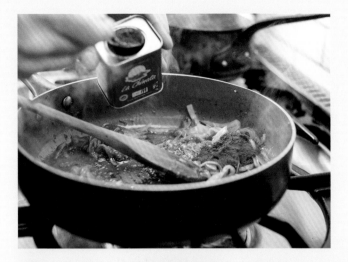

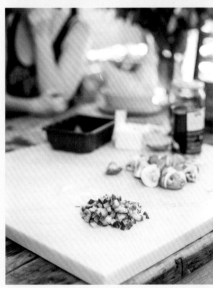

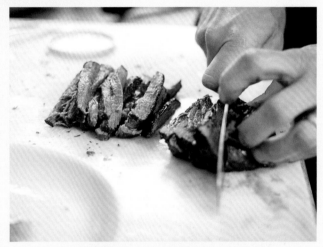

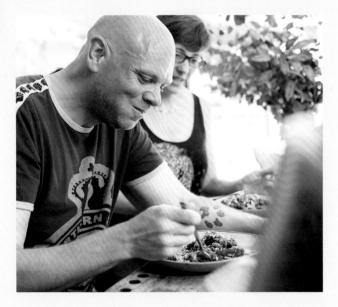

Asian beef with pak choi and radishes

Packed with some of my favourite Asian flavours, this is delicious and satisfying. Rich, savoury and yet so simple to make, it seems more like a take-away treat. Just don't add rice!

Serves: 2

Carb count: 26g per person

2 rib eye steaks (about 250g each)
Vegetable oil, for cooking
6 garlic cloves, sliced
4cm knob of fresh ginger, finely diced
2 tsp cracked black pepper
1 tbsp Chinese five-spice powder
2 star anise
2 tsp clear honey
75ml dark soy sauce
75ml rice wine vinegar
75ml white wine
150ml chicken gravy (I make it with Bisto chicken gravy granules)
2 heads of pak choi, leaves separated
¼ white radish, also called mooli or daikon (about 80g), peeled and cut into julienne
A bunch of breakfast radishes, topped and halved lengthways
½ bunch of spring onions, trimmed and chopped into 2cm pieces
1 red chilli, thinly sliced, seeds and all
A little sesame oil
Sea salt and freshly ground black pepper

1 Season the steaks on both sides with salt and pepper. Heat a large, heavy-bottomed frying pan or sauté pan over a medium-high heat and add a splash of oil. Place the steaks in the pan. Cook them until nicely browned on both sides, allowing about 3 minutes each side for medium-rare. Remove the steaks from the pan and place on a warm plate. Set aside to rest.

2 Add a little more oil to the pan, followed by the garlic and ginger. Cook quite rapidly, stirring, until lightly golden – be very careful not to burn them. Stir in the cracked pepper, five-spice powder and star anise.

3 Add the honey and cook until it darkens to a rich, caramel colour. Pour in the soy sauce, which will stop the cooking, then add the rice wine vinegar and wine. Bring to the boil and let bubble to reduce by two-thirds.

4 Add the gravy and bring to the boil. Turn the heat down to a simmer and stir in the pak choi and all the radishes. Cook until the leaves are just wilted, then add the spring onions and chilli. Season with salt and pepper and add a trickle of sesame oil.

5 Cut the rested steak into slices, about 1cm thick. Pile the vegetables into warmed shallow bowls. Place the beef slices alongside and pour over the liquor, then serve.

The Dope: Cooked quickly, <u>pak choi</u> adds great crunch and leafy vitality to soups, broths and stews.

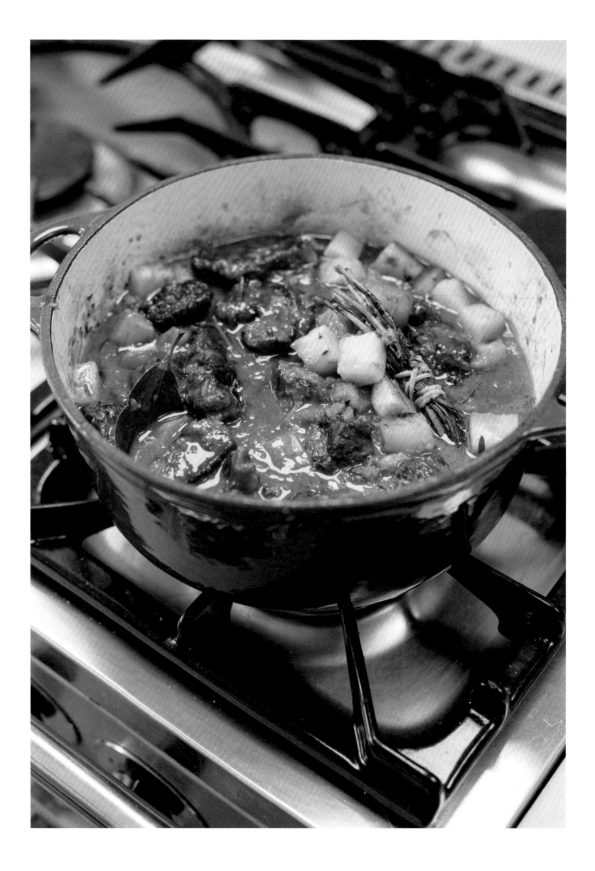

Braised beef with horseradish

I've swapped the carb-heavy potatoes and carrots typically found in a beef stew for turnips and kohlrabi. These low-carb vegetables have a peppery taste, which works really well with the fresh, fiery horseradish.

Serves: 6

Carb count: 29g per person

Vegetable oil, for cooking
1.2kg shin of beef, cut into
   3cm pieces
2 onions, finely diced
4cm knob of fresh ginger, grated
2 celery sticks, tough strings
   removed, diced
6 bay leaves
A bunch of rosemary (about 6–8
   sprigs), tied with kitchen string
750ml beef stock
200g button mushrooms, stalks
   removed
30g horseradish, peeled and
   freshly grated
4 turnips, peeled and cut into
   3cm chunks
2 kohlrabi, peeled and cut into
   3cm chunks
2 tbsp beef gravy granules (I use
   Bisto), optional
2 tbsp English mustard
Sea salt and freshly ground
   black pepper

1 Place a large, lidded flameproof casserole over a medium heat and add a thin film of oil. Season the beef and fry, in batches, until well browned and crisp all over; don't crowd the pan or the pieces will steam rather than brown. Transfer the browned meat to a plate to rest.

2 Preheat the oven to 150°C/Fan 130°C/Gas 2. Turn the heat down under the casserole to medium-low and add the onions and ginger. Sweat gently, stirring occasionally, for about 10–15 minutes until softened. Add the celery and cook for a further 2–3 minutes, then add the bay leaves and rosemary and give it a good stir.

3 Return the beef to the casserole, along with any juices that have accumulated on the plate. Pour in the stock and bring to the boil, then stir in the mushrooms and horseradish. Turn the heat down to a simmer and season with some salt and pepper. Put the lid on and cook in the oven for 2 hours.

4 Take out the casserole and stir in the turnips and kohlrabi. Return to the oven, without the lid, and cook for a further hour. The sauce will reduce and thicken slightly and the beef will become very tender. If you think the sauce needs thickening, stir in the gravy granules.

5 Finally, stir in the mustard and check the seasoning. Serve in warmed bowls.

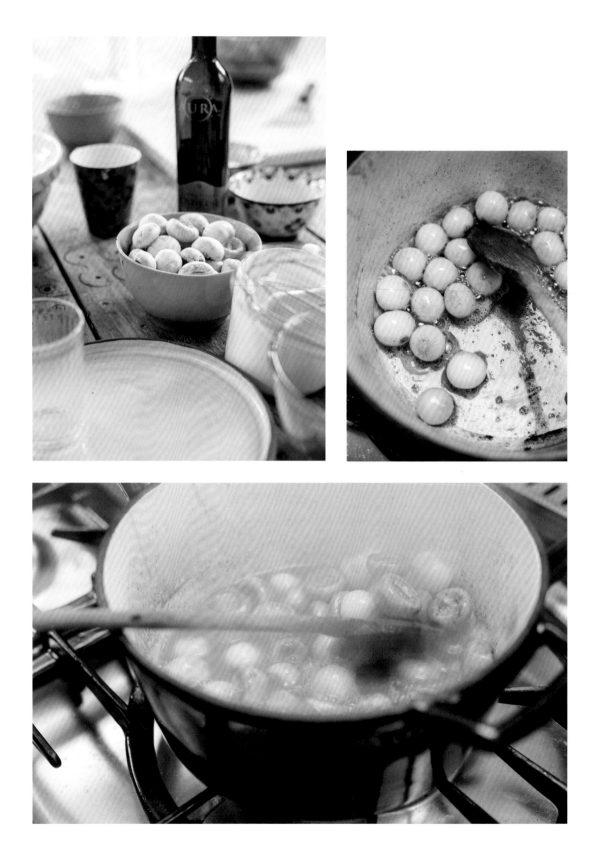

Blanquette of pork with celeriac spaghetti

This is my play on the elegant and sophisticated French dish, *blanquette de veau*. It's traditionally made with veal and served with rice but I find celeriac spaghetti works beautifully with my pork version, and the lovely aniseed flavour from the tarragon lifts the whole dish.

Serves: 4–6
Carb count: 13–9g per person

1kg shoulder of pork, skinned and cut into large bite-sized pieces
6 garlic cloves, peeled
2 chicken stock cubes
1 tbsp black peppercorns
2 star anise
2 cloves
A bunch of rosemary (about 7–8 sprigs), tied with kitchen string
100g butter
250g baby onions
250g button mushrooms, stalks removed
250ml double cream
1 tbsp Dijon mustard
2 free-range eggs
2 tbsp crème fraîche
1 celeriac, peeled (about 800g prepared weight)
4 tbsp chopped tarragon
Sea salt and freshly ground black pepper

1 Preheat the oven to 150°C/Fan 130°C/Gas 2. Put the pork pieces in a large saucepan and pour on enough cold water to cover. Bring to the boil and skim off any scum from the surface. Drain the pork in a colander and rinse under cold running water.

2 Put the pork into a flameproof casserole. Add the whole garlic cloves, pour in 1 litre water and crumble in the stock cubes. Tie the peppercorns, star anise and cloves in a piece of muslin with kitchen string. Drop the bundle into the pan, along with the rosemary. Bring to the boil, then put the lid on. Cook in the oven for 2 hours. Take out the casserole and leave to rest for 30 minutes.

3 Remove and discard the rosemary and muslin spice bag. Drain the pork and garlic cloves in a colander set over a large bowl; reserve the cooking liquor.

4 Put the casserole back on the hob. Add 50g of the butter and melt over a medium heat, then tip in the onions and sauté, shaking the pan frequently, until they are a nice golden colour. This should take about 8–10 minutes. Add the mushrooms and cook for a further 5–6 minutes, stirring from time to time, until most of their liquid has evaporated.

Continues overleaf →

Continued from previous page ➜

⑤ Add a ladleful or two of the reserved liquor to the pan and reduce to a glaze. Add the double cream and bring to the boil. Stir in the mustard, then simmer to reduce the sauce by half. Return the pork to the casserole, stir and reduce the heat to low.

⑥ While the sauce is simmering, whisk the eggs and crème fraîche together in a bowl; set aside. Using a spiralizer, turn the celeriac into spaghetti.

⑦ Melt the remaining butter in a saucepan over a medium-high heat. Add a splash of water and some salt and pepper and bring to the boil. Tip in the celeriac spaghetti and cook until just softened, 4–5 minutes.

⑧ Pour the creamy egg mix into the casserole, stirring as you do so. Cook over a very low heat, stirring constantly, for 4–5 minutes until the sauce thickens; don't let it simmer or the eggs will curdle. If it becomes too thick, add a little more of the pork cooking liquor. Season with salt and pepper, then take off the heat and stir in the chopped tarragon.

⑨ Divide the celeriac spaghetti between warmed plates and spoon the blanquette of pork on top. Serve immediately.

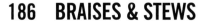

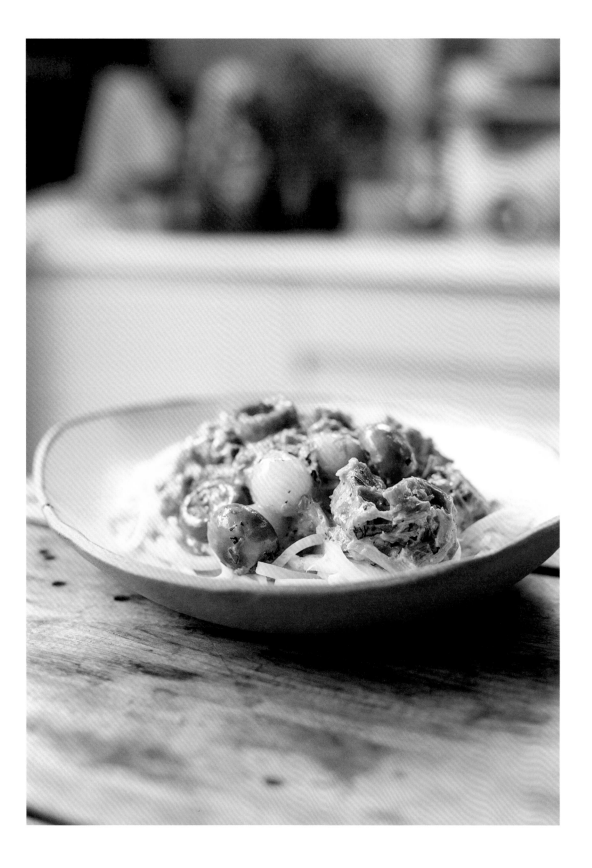

Chinese pork hot pot

This is a really nourishing dish – full of warming flavours and enticing aromatics, it makes the kitchen smell fantastic! I use pork belly here, but it's a good way of using leftover roast meat too. Duck, beef, chicken or even lamb all work very well.

Serves: 4

Carb count: 18g per person

800g piece of boned pork belly, skin scored
1 tbsp plus 2 tsp Szechuan peppercorns
4 star anise
3–4 tbsp vegetable oil
4 dried red chillies
8 garlic cloves, grated
7cm knob of fresh ginger, chopped
Finely pared zest of ½ orange
2 chicken stock cubes
2 tbsp Sriracha sauce
300g shiitake mushrooms
2 fresh red chillies, chopped, seeds and all
1 head of Chinese leaf, cut into 4cm pieces
2 bunches of spring onions, trimmed and cut into 2cm lengths

1 Preheat the oven to 150°C/Fan 130°C/Gas 2. Place the pork belly, skin side up, on a wire rack over a roasting tin and roast in the oven for 2½–3 hours, or until the skin is crisp and golden brown. Set aside to rest for at least 30 minutes.

2 Remove the skin from the pork belly and, if you like crackling, puff it up under a hot grill; reserve for serving. Cut the meat into chunks.

3 Tie the Szechuan peppercorns and star anise in a piece of muslin, using kitchen string, to form a bundle.

4 Heat a large, heavy-bottomed saucepan over a medium-high heat. Add the oil, then the muslin spice bundle and dried chillies. Fry, stirring, for 1–2 minutes until very fragrant and then stir in the garlic, ginger and orange zest. Cook, stirring, for 1–2 minutes.

5 Crumble in the stock cubes and add the Sriracha sauce then pour on 1 litre water. Bring to the boil, then add the mushrooms and fresh chillies. Lower the heat and simmer for 15 minutes. Remove the spice bundle and simmer for a further 10–15 minutes.

6 Add the pork and warm through. Stir in the Chinese leaf and spring onions and cook for a minute or two until wilted. Serve in warmed bowls, topped with some crackling if you like.

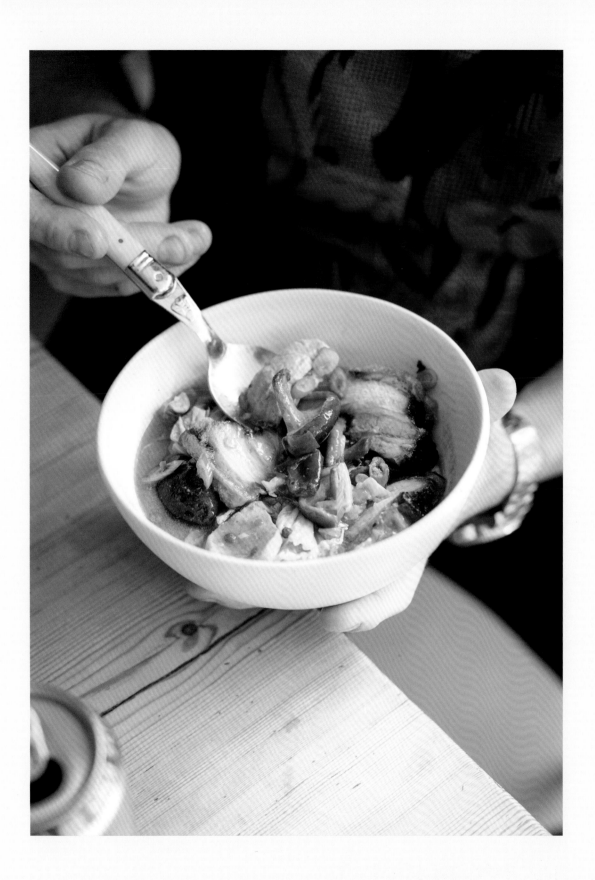

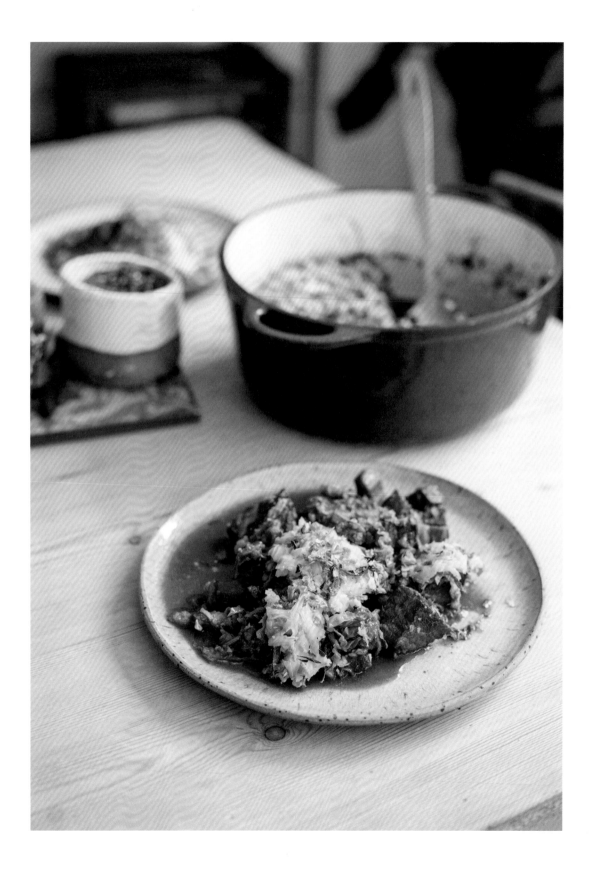

Pork stew with a smoked cheese crust

I've found pork really useful while following my low-carb regime, as it's so versatile and has great texture. Finishing this stew with a cheesy, crunchy topping makes it a brilliant one-dish dinner.

Serves: 4–6

Carb count: 21–14g per person

Vegetable oil, for cooking
1kg shoulder of pork, skin
    removed, cut into 3cm cubes
200g pancetta, diced
2 onions, halved and sliced
10 garlic cloves, grated
2 chicken stock cubes
200ml white wine
2 tsp cracked black pepper
A bunch of rosemary (about
    6–8 sprigs), tied together
    with kitchen string
400ml chicken stock
3 tbsp medium-hot German mustard
1 Savoy cabbage, cored and finely
    sliced
2 x 70g packets of pork
    scratchings, packets bashed
    to coarsely crush
6 tbsp dried onion flakes
3 tbsp thyme leaves
250g smoked cheese, grated
Sea salt and freshly ground
    black pepper

1 Set a large, lidded, heavy flameproof casserole over a medium heat. Add a little oil and sauté the pork in batches until golden brown. Remove with a slotted spoon; drain on kitchen paper.

2 Add the pancetta to the casserole and fry until it has rendered plenty of its fat and is lightly browned. Reduce the heat slightly and add the onions and garlic. Sweat gently, stirring occasionally, for 10–15 minutes until softened.

3 Crumble in the stock cubes, then add the wine and cracked black pepper. Bring to the boil and simmer until the liquor is reduced down to a rich glaze. Meanwhile, preheat the oven to 150°C/Fan 130°C/Gas 2.

4 Return the pork to the casserole, add the herb bundle and pour on the stock. Bring to the boil, put the lid on and cook in the oven for 2 hours.

5 Stir in the mustard and some salt and pepper. Spread the sliced cabbage over the pork. Cover and cook in the oven for a further 45 minutes. Remove the lid and return to the oven for a further 15–20 minutes to reduce the liquor.

6 In a small bowl, mix the pork scratchings with the onion flakes and thyme leaves. Take out the casserole and scatter the cheese over the surface, followed by the crunchy pork mixture. Return to the oven for a further 25–30 minutes. Leave to stand for 5 minutes before serving.

Easy sauerkraut with sausages and bacon

This tasty and comforting dish is based on *choucroute garni*, a favourite from the Alsace region of France. Pickled cabbage, or sauerkraut, is enjoying a bit of a revival at the moment as we begin to understand how beneficial fermented foods can be for our health. It's fairly easy to track down jars of good-quality sauerkraut in shops, delis and markets, and few things are better with some great pork sausages.

Serves: 6–8

Carb count: 11–8g per person

2 tsp white peppercorns
1 tsp juniper berries
6 cloves
Vegetable oil, for cooking
2 onions, halved and sliced
4 garlic cloves, grated
650g ready-made sauerkraut
3 tbsp freshly grated horseradish
300ml white wine
4 bay leaves
1 chicken stock cube
2 tbsp yellow mustard seeds
500g thick-cut garlic sausage,
    such as Polish kielbasa
10 best-quality frankfurters
6 thick slices of streaky bacon,
    cut 2cm thick (ask your butcher
    for these)
Flaky sea salt

To serve:
A handful of flat-leaf parsley,
    leaves picked from stems
A selection of mustards

1 First, tie the peppercorns, juniper and cloves in a piece of muslin, using kitchen string.

2 Preheat the oven to 160°C/Fan 140°C/Gas 3. Warm a splash of oil in a large flameproof casserole over a medium-low heat. Add the onions and garlic and sweat gently, stirring from time to time, for about 10–15 minutes until softened.

3 Add the sauerkraut, along with the grated horseradish and muslin spice bag. Pour on the wine and 100ml water. Add the bay leaves, crumble in the stock cube and stir in the mustard seeds. Bring to the boil, then add the garlic sausage, frankfurters and bacon.

4 Turn the heat down to a simmer. Put the lid on the casserole and place in the oven. Cook for 1½ hours, then remove from the oven and season with flaky sea salt.

5 Serve on warmed plates, scattered with the parsley, with a choice of mustards on the side.

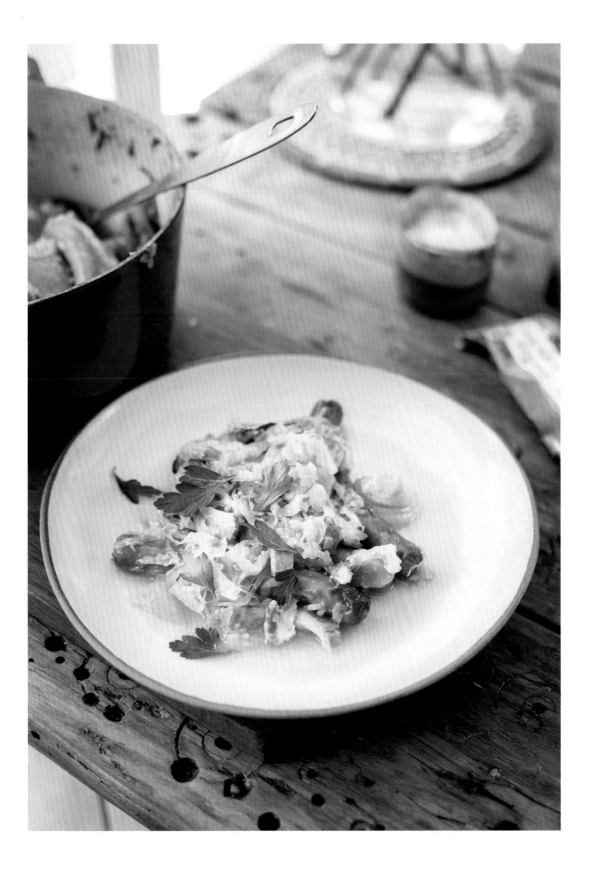

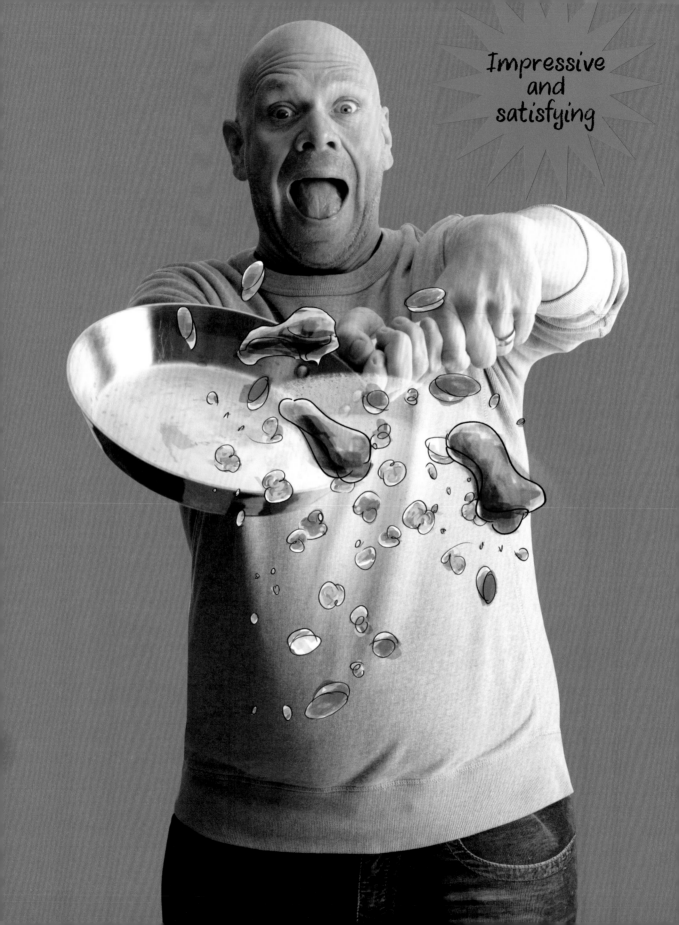

Impressive
and
satisfying

PAN-FRYING & ROASTS

'VE THROWN THE WHOLE SPICE DRAWER at this chapter – pepper, chilli, cumin, coriander, mustard seeds, paprika, turmeric, cinnamon and cayenne – all of the things I love. In sizeable quantities they can give you a dopamine boost, but, more importantly, they make things taste great.

One of my favourite things about roasting meat and fish rather than using other cooking methods is that you have the chance to experiment with dry spice rubs. These impart incredible flavour and help to create a beautiful, tasty crust. In the quest to banish bland diet food, a great spice rub is a real asset.

Some of the dishes in this chapter, such as the spiced leg of lamb (page 218) and Indian spiced goose (page 210) are roasted slowly in the oven. Here, it's a similar principle to the braises and stews in the previous chapter, with the flavour intensifying in a fantastic way. This is some of the nicest food you're ever going to eat and it certainly won't make you feel you're on a diet. Tuck into a roast shoulder of pork with rhubarb (page 228) or pulled shoulder of lamb with mint gravy (page 213) and you'll see what I mean.

But it doesn't all have to be slow. For those evenings when you don't have much time, pan-frying is a great short cut to flavour. Try Cumberland sausages with onion gravy (page 233) or the rib eye steak chasseur (page 220) if you want a relatively quick and satisfying meal. Or if you want something more refined, try the sea bass with champagne and vanilla sauce (page 200) – it has a touch of Michelin-starred luxury about it but it's not at all difficult to put together. Also, the smell of vanilla has been linked to the release of feel-good endorphins, so that's a win-win dinner result.

Marrying combinations of flavours is one of the most exciting things about my job. You'll find that many of the side dishes in this book can be bumped up into main courses in their own right too. No one wants to – or should – eat meat every single day, so from time to time, ditch the meat and focus on the veg. Throughout this book, I've tried to create intense flavour and great texture wherever I can. This certainly goes for every single one of the main dishes in this book, but I've also put a lot of thought into the side dishes too (see opposite).

Cracking side dishes

Here are some favourite sides that you might like to try, even if you don't make the 'main' recipe they feature in:

* Cauliflower couscous (pages 155 and 166). You can customise this according to the herbs and spices you have to hand. It's great with simply grilled meat or fish, or served on its own as a main course salad.

* Creamed spinach (page 233). This tastes luxuriously creamy and goes with all kinds of grilled meat and fish.

* Broccoli and frankfurters (page 225). Ideal for a quick tea – grate some cheese over the top and pop it under the grill if you want to make it a bit more substantial.

* Mustard-glazed greens (page 214). This is one of my favourite go-to quick sides. It goes with pretty much any main course and works brilliantly with turnip tops too.

* Coconut and apple salad (page 219). Refreshing, crunchy and tasty, this is lovely on its own or with any hot, fiery barbecue.

* Red cabbage salad (page 222). I like this simple combination of quick pickled cabbage and white radish with everything from grilled, roasted or barbecued meats to oily fish such as sardines or mackerel.

197

Soy-glazed cod with chilli, garlic and ginger

Fish is always a great choice when you want a lighter meal, but I promise the big, powerful flavours of this dish will leave you feeling more than satisfied. So that everything's ready at the same time, get cracking on the onion salad when you've put the cod in the oven. Pollock, hake and haddock also work well in this dish – just buy the best and freshest fish you can find.

Serves: 2

Carb count: 46g per person

For the fish:

2 skinless, boneless cod fillets (about 200g each)

Finely grated zest and juice of 2 limes

4 tbsp dark soy sauce

3 garlic cloves, crushed

3cm knob of fresh ginger, grated

2 tbsp mushroom ketchup (I like Geo Watkins)

1 tbsp Sriracha sauce

1 tbsp clear honey

2 tbsp sesame seeds, toasted in a dry frying pan until fragrant and golden

2 large red chillies, thinly sliced, seeds and all

For the onion and fennel salad:

2 red onions, halved and thinly sliced

2 white onions, halved and thinly sliced

1 fennel bulb, halved and cut into thin strips

1 tbsp flaky sea salt

A bunch of spring onions, trimmed and finely sliced

A bunch of coriander (about 25g), leaves picked from stems

2 tbsp rice wine vinegar

2 tbsp sesame oil

① To prepare the fish, mix together the lime zest and juice, soy sauce, garlic, ginger, mushroom ketchup, Sriracha sauce and honey in a bowl. Place the cod in the bowl and turn to coat in the mixture. Cover and leave the cod fillets to marinate in the fridge for 2 hours.

② Preheat the oven to 200°C/Fan 180°C/Gas 6. Place the cod fillets in a roasting tin and spoon on the marinade. Bake for 20–25 minutes, basting the fillets with the marinade every 5 minutes. The liquor will reduce to a beautiful glaze covering the cod.

③ Once the cod is in the oven, prepare the salad. Put the sliced red and white onions and the fennel strips into a bowl and toss with the salt. Leave to soften for 10 minutes, then tip into a colander and rinse under cold running water. Pat dry with a clean tea towel or kitchen paper and transfer to a bowl.

④ Add the spring onions and coriander to the salad and toss well. Just before serving, dress with the rice wine vinegar and sesame oil.

⑤ When the roasted cod is ready, place on warmed plates and sprinkle with the toasted sesame seeds and sliced chillies. Pile the onion and fennel salad alongside and serve.

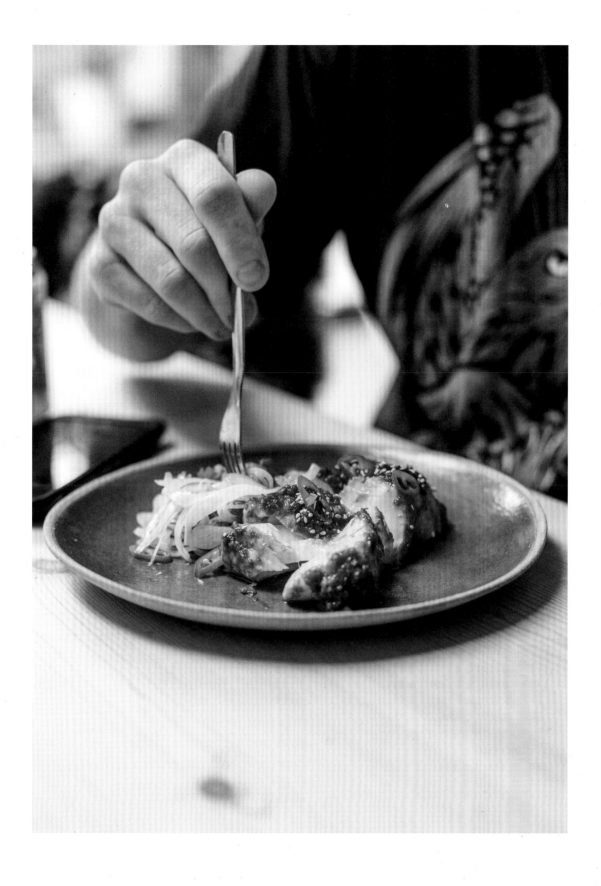

Sea bass with champagne and vanilla sauce

If you are looking for something special, this elegant, light dish hits the spot. Adding vanilla to a sauce for fish is a fine dining classic, but here there is an added bonus – it helps promote the release of feel-good endorphins.

Serves: 2

Carb count: 17g per person

2 sea bass fillets (about 200g
    each), skin on and pin-boned
Vegetable oil, for cooking
50g coconut flour
50g butter
Juice of 1 lemon
Sea salt and freshly ground
    white pepper

For the fennel:
40ml best-quality extra virgin
    olive oil, plus extra to finish
1 small onion, finely diced
1 large fennel bulb, trimmed and
    finely diced
2 garlic cloves, grated
1 tbsp mustard seeds, toasted in
    a dry frying pan until they pop
1 tsp Dijon mustard
A small handful of dill, chopped

For the sauce:
Extra virgin olive oil, for cooking
2 banana shallots, finely diced
150ml champagne or sparkling
    wine
1 vanilla pod, split lengthways,
    seeds scraped out
100ml double cream
75g butter, chilled and cut
    into cubes
Lemon juice, to taste

1 For the fennel, warm the olive oil in a large saucepan over a medium-low heat. Add the onion, fennel and garlic and sauté gently for about 12–15 minutes until softened. Remove from the heat and stir in the mustard seeds, mustard and dill. Season with salt and pepper.

2 To make the sauce, warm a splash of olive oil in a saucepan over a medium-low heat. Add the shallots and sauté for about 10 minutes, until softened. Pour in the wine and add the vanilla seeds and empty pod. Increase the heat, bring to the boil and reduce to a glaze. Add the cream and reduce by half. Turn the heat to low and whisk in the butter, a cube at a time, ensuring each is fully incorporated before adding the next. Remove the vanilla pod and season with salt, pepper and lemon juice to taste. Set aside; keep warm.

3 To cook the fish, warm a large non-stick frying pan over a medium heat and add a little oil. Dust the skin side of the fish with the coconut flour. Place in the pan, skin side down and fry, without moving, for about 4 minutes, until the skin is crisp and the fish is cooked 80 per cent of the way through. Flip the fish over, add the butter and lemon juice and baste the fish for a minute or two, until just cooked. Season.

4 Spoon the sauce onto warmed plates. Top with the fish and fennel and add a drizzle of olive oil.

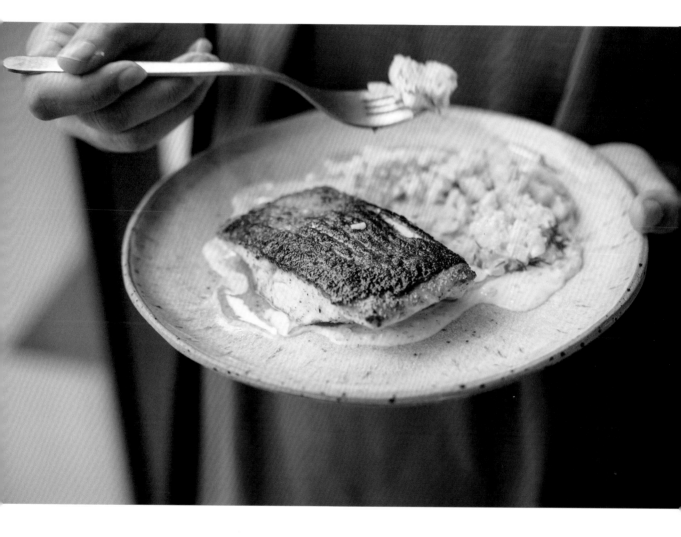

Roast chicken with hazelnut pesto

I like to slow-roast chicken to keep it moist and tender, and to serve it with lightly pickled mushrooms and asparagus, when it is in season. It's worth making this for two (just scale down the veg accordingly) as it's always great to have some leftover roast chicken in the fridge for quick salads and packed lunches. The aromatic herby pesto is delicious with the chicken, whether you're serving it hot or cold.

Serves: 4

Carb count: 7g per person

1 free-range chicken (about 1.4kg)
Vegetable oil, for cooking
1 chicken stock cube
Sea salt and freshly ground
    black pepper

For the pesto:
100g hazelnuts
A large bunch of basil (about 100g),
    leaves picked from stems
50g Parmesan cheese, freshly
    grated
1 garlic clove, grated
50–100ml good-quality extra virgin
    olive oil
Finely grated zest of 1 lemon

For the vegetables:
400g chestnut mushrooms, stems
    removed
2 tbsp flaky sea salt
3 tbsp sherry vinegar
1½ tbsp truffle oil
2 bunches of asparagus (each
    8–10 spears)
100g butter

1 First toast the hazelnuts for the pesto: preheat the oven to 200°C/Fan 180°C/Gas 6. Scatter the nuts on an oven tray and toast in the oven for 5–6 minutes, until fragrant and the skins are blistered; watch carefully as they can quickly burn. Wrap the nuts in a clean tea towel and leave for 5 minutes, then rub vigorously in the tea towel to remove the papery skins. Let cool.

2 Reduce the oven temperature to 140°C/Fan 120°C/Gas 1. Place the chicken in a roasting tray and drizzle with a little oil, then crumble over the stock cube to give it a good, even dusting. Roast in the oven for 2½ hours.

3 Turn the oven up to 220°C/Fan 200°C/Gas 7 and continue to roast the chicken for a further 20 minutes, until the skin crisps and colours. Remove and leave to rest for 20 minutes.

4 Make the pesto while the chicken is roasting. Place the cooled, toasted hazelnuts in a food processor and blitz to a rough powder. Add the basil, Parmesan and garlic and pulse to blend. Slowly pour in the olive oil, pulsing as you go, adding just enough to give the texture you like. Add the lemon zest and season

Continues overleaf →

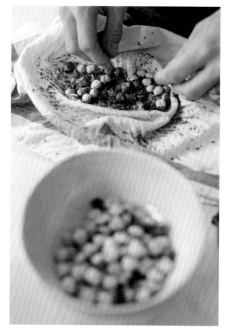
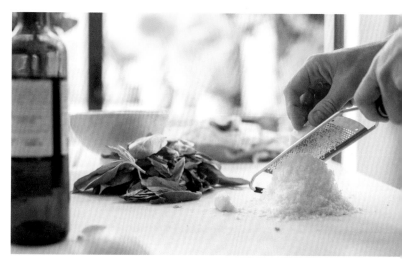
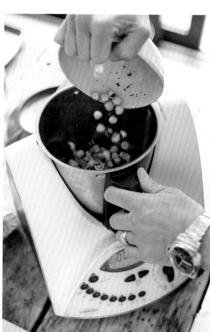
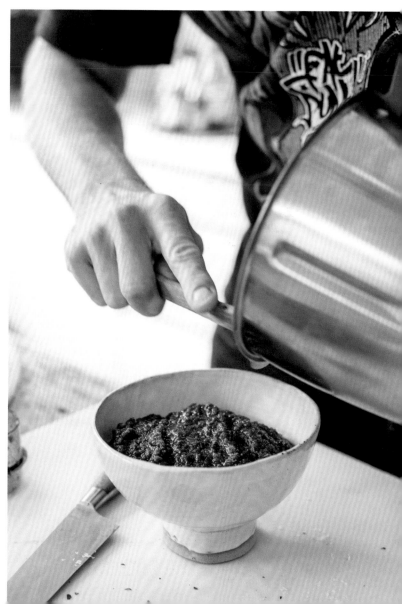

Continued from previous page →

to taste with salt and pepper. Transfer to a container, seal and refrigerate until needed. If you don't use all of the pesto, it will keep for a day or so in the fridge, if you cover the surface with a film of olive oil.

5 Also prepare the vegetables while the chicken is in the oven. Slice the mushrooms as thinly as possible. Place in a bowl, sprinkle with the flaky salt and toss to mix. Leave to stand for 5 minutes. Tip the mushrooms into a colander and rinse briefly under the cold tap, then pat dry on a clean tea towel or kitchen paper. Place the mushrooms in a bowl, add the sherry vinegar and truffle oil and toss to mix.

6 To prepare the asparagus, cut off the woody ends and peel the lower part of the spears with a vegetable peeler. In a large sauté pan, bring 200ml water to a simmer. Add the butter and some salt and pepper. Lower in the asparagus and cook, turning, until the stems are just tender when pierced with a small, sharp knife.

7 Carve the rested chicken and serve with the lightly pickled mushrooms, tender asparagus and hazelnut pesto.

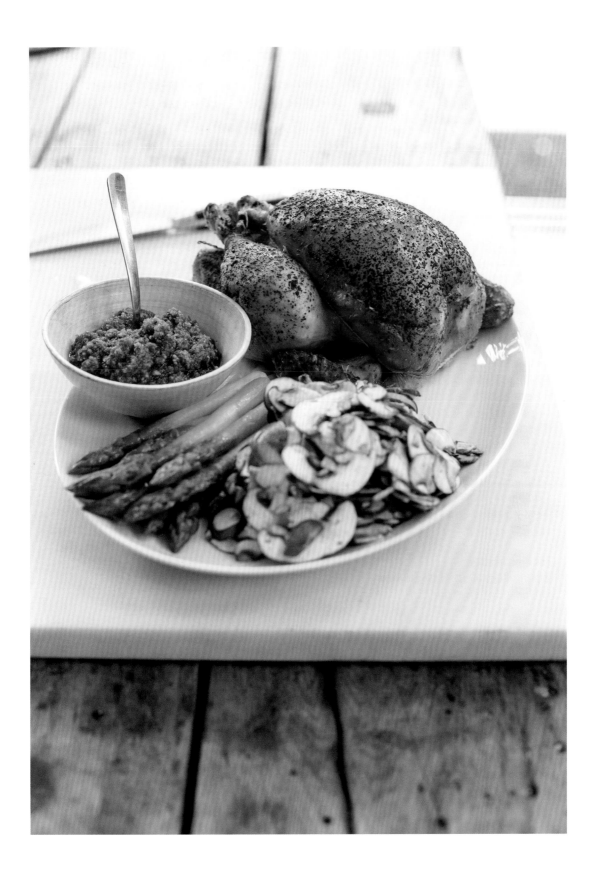

Piri piri chicken with Little Gem salad

I'll tell you a secret. I once had an in-depth conversation with a fellow Michelin-starred chef about just how good Nando's extra hot chicken is. Who doesn't love piri piri chicken? This is such a great recipe, a real favourite of mine for when that hot, hot chicken craving hits. The crisp, cool, herby salad is really all you need with it.

Serves: 4

Carb count: 10g per person

1 large free-range chicken (about 2kg)

For the chilli paste:
2 dried hot red chillies
100ml red wine vinegar
6 fresh red chillies, roughly chopped, seeds and all
6 garlic cloves, peeled
2 tsp flaky sea salt
2 tsp smoked paprika
1 tsp dried oregano
1 tsp dried thyme
1 tsp erythritol (sugar replacement)
Juice of 2 lemons

For the salad:
2 Little Gem lettuces, leaves separated from the core
½ cucumber, halved, deseeded and sliced
6 pickled green chillies, roughly chopped
½ bunch of mint (about 15g), leaves picked from stems
½ bunch of coriander (about 15g), leaves picked from the stems
2 tbsp salad cream
Sea salt and freshly ground black pepper

① Remove the skin from the chicken: work your fingers under the skin, over the flesh, until you have loosened it enough to pull it off. Score the chicken all over (including the legs and the underside), making the cuts about 1cm deep.

② To prepare the chilli paste, put the dried chillies in a small saucepan with the wine vinegar and bring to the boil. Remove from the heat and leave to cool and allow the chillies to rehydrate.

③ Put the fresh chillies, garlic and rehydrated chillies and their soaking vinegar into a food processor and blitz. Add the salt, smoked paprika, oregano, thyme, erythritol and lemon juice and blitz again to a paste.

④ Spread the paste all over the chicken and massage it into the cuts (protect your hands with latex gloves or wash them thoroughly after handling the chilli paste). Place the chicken in a roasting tin, cover with cling film and put into the fridge. Leave to marinate for at least 4 hours, but overnight would be even better to allow the flavours to develop.

⑤ Preheat the oven to 140°C/Fan 120°C/Gas 1. Unwrap the chicken and cook in the oven for 2½ hours.

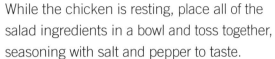

6 Turn the oven setting up to 220°C/Fan 200°C/ Gas 7 and cook for a further 25–30 minutes, until a golden crust forms on the outside of the chicken. Remove from the oven and set aside to rest for 20 minutes.

7 While the chicken is resting, place all of the salad ingredients in a bowl and toss together, seasoning with salt and pepper to taste.

8 Carve the rested chicken and serve with the salad. It is also good served cold.

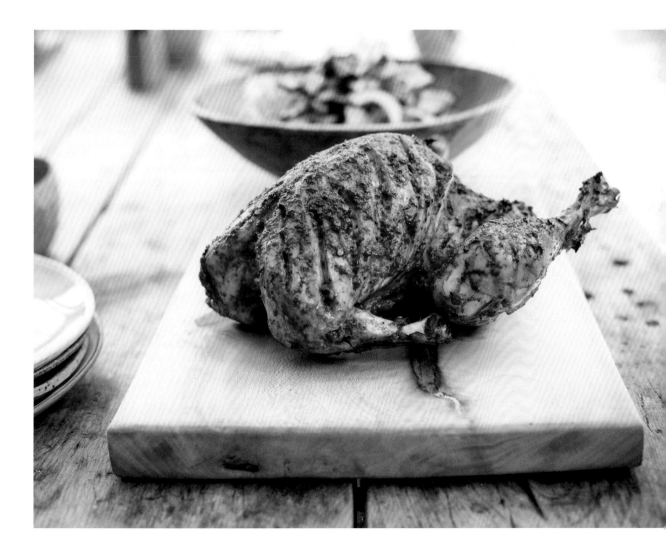

Turkey schnitzel with lemon and caper butter

This is full of great flavours – the sort of thing you might find in a smart French brasserie. Feel free to use a different white meat, but I've opted for turkey because it's high in dopamine-releasing amino acids. Parmesan, sesame seeds and onion flakes take the place of the usual breadcrumb crust.

Serves: 2

Carb count: 15g per person

2 free-range skinless turkey
   breast fillets (about 200g each)
100ml buttermilk
40g Parmesan cheese, grated
30g dried onion flakes
30g coconut flour
20g sesame seeds
2 free-range egg yolks
40ml milk
Vegetable oil, for cooking
100g butter
Finely grated zest of 1 lemon,
   plus some of the juice
2 tbsp capers
2 tbsp chopped parsley
2 free-range duck eggs
4 anchovy fillets in oil, drained
Sea salt and freshly ground
   black pepper

To serve (optional):
Gherkins, green pickled chillies
   and marinated artichokes

1 One at a time, bash the turkey fillets between two sheets of cling film with a rolling pin to flatten to an even thickness.

2 Place the turkey breasts in a bowl with the buttermilk and leave to tenderise for at least 2 hours, or in the fridge overnight.

3 For the coating, mix the grated Parmesan, onion flakes, coconut flour and sesame seeds together in a bowl and season with salt and pepper. In a separate bowl, beat the egg yolks with the milk.

4 Dip the turkey fillets into the egg mix and then into the coating, turning to ensure they are covered all over. Warm a little oil in a non-stick frying pan over a medium heat. Add 40g of the butter and let it melt and turn golden brown. Fry the turkey fillets, one at a time, on both sides until browned and crisp. Set aside; keep warm.

5 Melt the remaining butter in the pan and cook to a rich golden brown (the noisette stage); don't let it burn. Add about 1 tbsp of the lemon juice, taste and add more if you would like the sauce a little sharper. Add the capers and lemon zest. Season and stir in the chopped parsley.

6 Heat a splash of oil in a separate frying pan and carefully break in the duck eggs. Fry until the whites are set. Season with salt and pepper to taste.

7 Place the turkey fillets on warmed plates and top with the fried duck eggs. Garnish with the anchovies and spoon on the sauce. Serve some gherkins, pickled chillies and marinated artichokes on the side if you like.

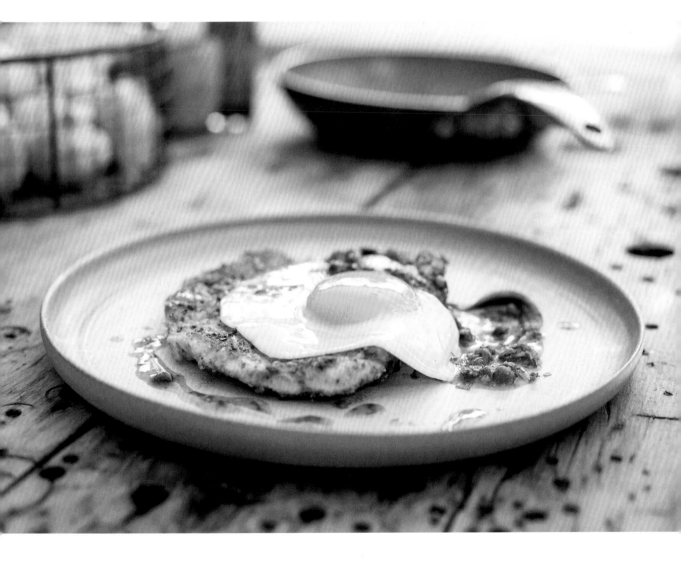

Indian spiced slow-roasted goose

Indian spices work brilliantly with dark poultry meat. The spicing is quite strong here, but the rich meat and the slow cooking pull everything together beautifully. Try it with duck too. This is a great dish to serve to a carb-loving crowd with heaps of rice and naan; just avoid them yourself and tuck into the spicy meat and greens.

Serves: 4–6

Carb count: 10–7g per person

1 free-range goose (about 5kg)
Finely grated zest and juice of
    2 limes
500ml chicken stock

For the spice blend:
1 tsp coriander seeds
1 tsp cumin seeds
1 tsp yellow mustard seeds
1 tsp cardamom pods
1 tsp black peppercorns
1 star anise
½ cinnamon stick
1 tsp chilli powder
1 tsp ground ginger
1 tsp garam masala

For the seasoned yoghurt:
200g wholemilk yoghurt
Finely grated zest and juice of
    1 lemon
1 garlic clove, grated
A pinch of sea salt
A small bunch of mint (about 15g),
    stems removed, leaves
    roughly chopped

For the greens:
75g butter
750g spring greens, cut into pieces
2 tsp dried chilli flakes
1 tsp sea salt

1 For the spice blend, in a frying pan over a medium heat, toast the coriander, cumin and mustard seeds, cardamom pods, black peppercorns, star anise and cinnamon stick until fragrant and lightly golden. Take the pan off the heat and stir in the chilli powder, ground ginger and garam masala. Tip into a bowl and leave to cool.

2 Preheat the oven to 150°C/Fan 130°C/Gas 2. Score the goose all over then place on a rack in a roasting tin. Grind the cooled spices to a powder, using a pestle and mortar or a spice grinder. Rub this all over the goose to coat.

3 Roast the goose for 4 hours, basting every half hour with its rendered fat. If it starts to brown too much, cover loosely with foil. To check it is cooked, pull the legs gently; they should give easily. Place the goose on a warm platter, scatter over the lime zest and cover loosely with foil. Leave to rest for 20 minutes.

4 Pour off the excess fat from the roasting tin. Place the tin on the hob over a medium-high heat. Add the lime juice and then pour in the stock. Bring to the boil, stirring with a wooden spoon and scraping up any brown bits stuck to the bottom of the tin. Simmer to reduce by two-thirds, to give you a lovely, spicy gravy.

5 Mix the yoghurt, lemon zest and juice, garlic and a pinch of salt together in a small bowl. Stir in the chopped mint and set aside.

6 To cook the greens, warm the butter in a large sauté pan or frying pan over a medium-high heat. When it stops foaming, add the spring greens with the chilli flakes and salt and toss over the heat until wilted.

7 Meanwhile, carve the goose from the bone. Serve with the wilted greens, gravy and some minted yoghurt on the side.

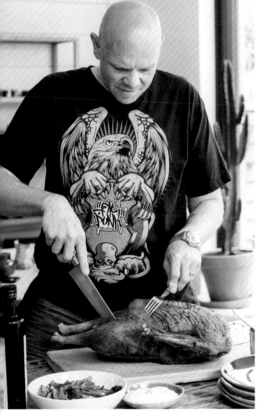

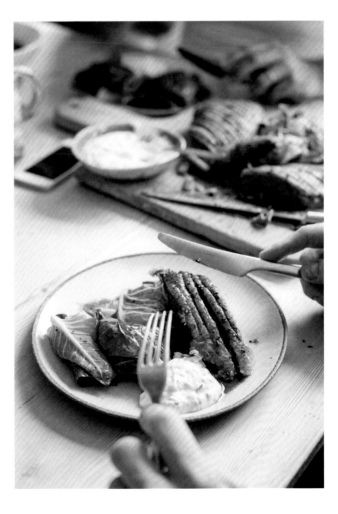

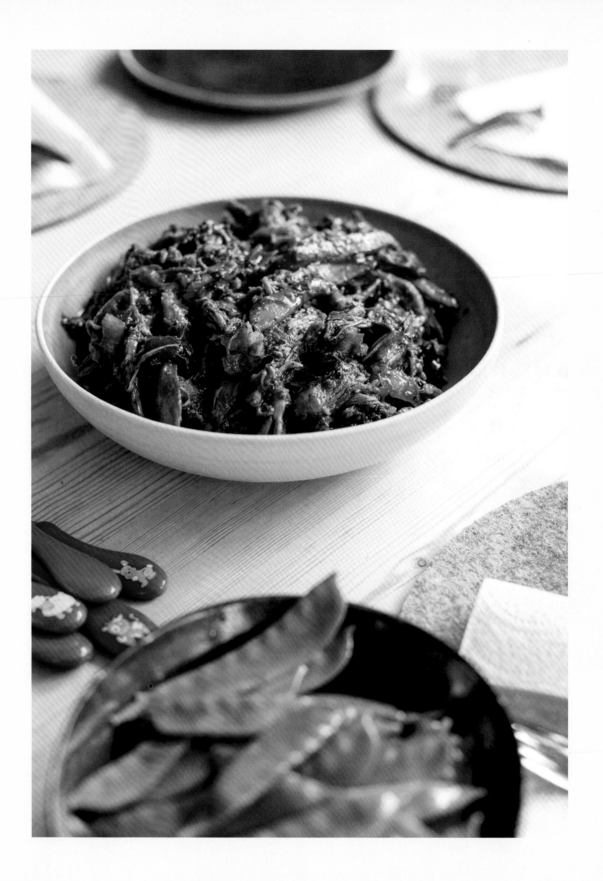

Pulled shoulder of lamb with mint gravy

This makes a wonderful dinner to share with friends, or you can serve it as part of a barbecue feast with lamb burgers or chops. It's great with any green veg or a salad, coleslaw (see pages 130 and 168) and some pickles.

Serves: 4–6

Carb count: 19–13g per person

1 shoulder of lamb (about 2.5kg), bone in

For the spice paste:
4 garlic cloves, grated
1 tbsp dried mint
2 tsp sea salt
2 tsp ground cinnamon
2 tsp ground cumin
1 tsp chilli powder
Finely grated zest and juice of 1 lemon
4 tbsp olive oil

For the mint gravy:
75g butter
2 onions, diced
1 tbsp tomato purée
100ml balsamic vinegar
3 x 400ml tins beef consommé (I like Campbell's)
100ml thick beef gravy (I make it with Bisto gravy granules), though you may not need this
A bunch of mint (about 30g), tough stems removed, leaves chopped
Sea salt and freshly ground black pepper

1 In a small bowl, mix the garlic, mint, salt and spices together. Add the lemon zest and juice and stir in the olive oil to form a paste.

2 Score the lamb shoulder deeply all over and then rub the spice paste all over the lamb and into the cuts. Place in a roasting tin and cover with cling film. Leave to marinate in the fridge for at least 4 hours, but preferably overnight.

3 Preheat the oven to 150°C/Fan 130°C/Gas 2. Remove the cling film from the lamb and roast for 4½–5 hours, until the meat flakes easily from the bone with a fork. Remove from the oven and leave to rest for 20 minutes.

4 Meanwhile, make the mint gravy. In a very large saucepan, warm the butter over a medium-low heat, add the onions and sweat gently for 10–15 minutes until softened, stirring occasionally. Stir in the tomato purée, then add the balsamic vinegar. Bring to the boil and let bubble to reduce to a glaze. Pour in the consommé and bring to the boil again. Lower the heat to a gentle simmer.

5 Flake the lamb from the bone and pull it apart with two forks. Add to the simmering stock and cook until the sauce thickens and coats the lamb. If the flavour needs a boost, add the beef gravy. Just before serving, stir in the chopped mint and taste for seasoning. Serve in warmed bowls.

Slow-roasted lamb with mustard-glazed greens

Shoulder of lamb has the perfect ratio of fat to meat for slow cooking, ensuring the meat stays wonderfully moist and tasty. The anchovy crust delivers a lovely salty, savoury flavour that works so well with the lamb, and the mustardy greens are an excellent accompaniment.

Serves: 4

Carb count: 13g per person

1 shoulder of lamb (about 2kg), bone in
10 garlic cloves, peeled
Sea salt and freshly ground black pepper

For the anchovy paste:
100g anchovy fillets in oil, drained and chopped
50g butter
½ tsp ground cinnamon
½ tsp ground mace
½ tsp ground white pepper
3 tbsp crushed pork scratchings

For the gravy:
3 banana shallots, cut into thin rings
150ml sherry vinegar
1 lamb stock cube
400ml ready-made lamb stock

For the greens:
75g butter, softened
2 heaped tbsp English mustard
1.2kg spring greens, cut into thick pieces
3 tbsp mustard seeds, toasted just until they begin to pop in a dry frying pan

1 Preheat the oven to 140°C/Fan 120°C/Gas 1. With a sharp knife, stab 10 deep holes in the lamb shoulder and push a peeled garlic clove into each one. Season with salt and pepper and place the lamb in a roasting tin. Cook for 4–5 hours, until the meat pulls away easily from the bone.

2 Meanwhile, make the anchovy paste. Using a pestle and mortar or mini food processor, work the anchovies, butter, cinnamon, mace and white pepper together to form a paste. Stir in the crushed pork scratchings.

3 Take the lamb from the oven and spread the anchovy paste all over it. Roast in the oven for a further 45 minutes–1 hour; it should just flake away from the bone. Lift the lamb onto a warmed platter and cover loosely with foil. Leave to rest for 30 minutes.

4 Meanwhile, make the gravy. Pour off the excess fat from the roasting tin, then place the tin on the hob over a medium heat. Add the shallots and cook until softened, stirring frequently, for about 10 minutes. Add the sherry vinegar and let bubble to reduce to a glaze. Crumble in the stock cube, pour in the stock and bring to the boil. Simmer to reduce by two-thirds to make a rich gravy.

To cook the greens, put 100ml water, the butter and mustard into a large saucepan and bring to the boil. Add some salt and pepper. Tip in the spring greens and stir around for a couple of minutes until just wilted. Stir in the mustard seeds.

Flake the lamb from the bone and serve with the gravy and mustard-glazed greens.

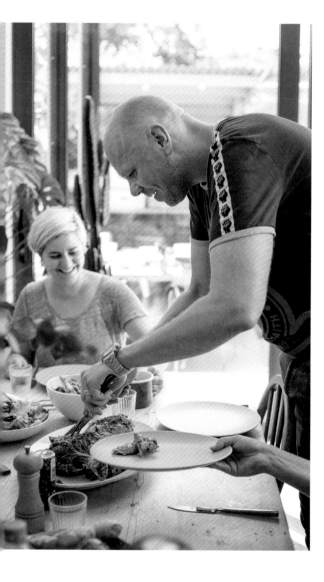

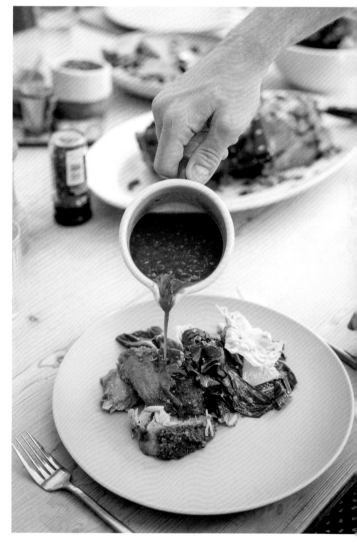

Roasted lamb rump with turnip top fricassée

I love the flavour of lamb rumps when they are heavily roasted on the outside but still pink in the middle, and they're great with peppery little turnips. When you're following a low-carb diet, turnip is such a brilliant vegetable. It has a potato-y structure, but it is lighter in density and has a more interesting flavour. The addition of the green turnip tops (known as *cima di rapa*) gives the fricassée a vibrant lift. If you can't get hold of them, used shredded kale or chopped spring greens instead.

Serves: 4

Carb count: 14g per person

For the lamb rumps:
2 tsp dried herbes de Provence
2 tbsp olive oil
4 lamb rumps (about 250g each), trimmed and scored
Vegetable oil, for cooking
Sea salt and freshly ground black pepper

For the turnip fricassée:
50g butter
2 onions, diced
2 garlic cloves, grated
1 green pepper, cored, deseeded and cut into 1cm dice
1 chicken stock cube
10 small (golf-ball-sized) turnips (about 60g each), peeled and halved
100ml double cream
2 tbsp crème fraîche
100g turnip tops or spring greens, roughly chopped
2 tbsp creamed horseradish

1 Preheat the oven to 180°C/Fan 160°C/Gas 4. Mix the dried herbs and olive oil together in a small bowl and then rub the mixture all over the lamb rumps. Season with salt and pepper.

2 Warm a large ovenproof frying pan over a medium heat and add the lamb rumps, skin side down. Render out as much fat as you can, but you may still need to add a splash more oil. When the skin is browned and crisp, turn the lamb rumps over and colour them on all sides.

3 Now place the pan in the oven and roast for 5–6 minutes until the rumps are medium-rare. Remove from the oven and leave to rest in the pan.

4 For the turnip fricassée, melt the butter in a large sauté pan over a medium-low heat. When it stops foaming, add the onions and garlic and sweat gently for 10–15 minutes until softened, stirring from time to time.

5 Stir in the green pepper, crumble in the stock cube and pour in 250ml water. Add the halved turnips, turn up the heat and bring to the boil. Cook until the liquid is reduced and the turnips are glazed and tender.

6 If the turnips are not quite cooked once the liquid is reduced, add a little more water and continue to cook until they are just soft.

7 Add the cream and crème fraîche, bring to the boil and let bubble to reduce down for 2–3 minutes. Stir in the turnip tops and creamed horseradish and cook for a minute or two, just until the greens have wilted.

8 Slice the lamb rumps, arrange on warmed plates and serve with the turnip fricassée.

The Dope: <u>Turnips</u> make a great low-carb alternative to potatoes for toppings to gratins or hot pots. Their peppery taste adds a welcome flavour boost too.

Spiced leg of lamb with cauliflower and coconut

I never tire of slow-roasted leg of lamb, but sometimes I like to experiment with old favourites. Here, I've ramped up the seasoning with a vindaloo-inspired spice rub. Marinating the meat overnight and then cooking it very slowly the following day enables the flavours to mingle and intensify in a delicious way. The pan-roasted cauliflower and crunchy, fresh coconut salad complement the rich, intense flavours of the meat brilliantly.

Serves: 6

Carb count: 21g per person

1 leg of lamb (about 2kg), bone in
Sea salt and freshly ground
   black pepper

For the spice paste:
1 tbsp cayenne pepper
1 tbsp ground coriander
1 tbsp cracked black pepper
1 tbsp yellow mustard seeds
½ tbsp ground cumin
½ tbsp ground turmeric
½ tbsp table salt
1 tsp ground ginger
1 tsp ground cinnamon
150ml distilled malt vinegar

For the cauliflower:
Vegetable oil, for cooking
2 cauliflowers (about 700g each),
   cut into florets
75ml distilled malt vinegar
2 tbsp cumin seeds, lightly
   toasted in a dry frying pan until
   just fragrant
250ml coconut cream

① For the spice paste, warm a dry frying pan over a medium-high heat, add all the spices and cook for a couple of minutes, stirring once or twice, until they are toasted and fragrant; be careful not to burn them. Tip into a bowl, stir in the vinegar and leave to cool.

② Make cuts all over the lamb and rub the spice paste all over the joint and into the cuts. Wrap in cling film and leave to marinate on a plate in the fridge for at least 8 hours or overnight.

③ Preheat the oven to 140°C/Fan 120°C/Gas 1. Take the lamb from the fridge and remove the cling film. Place the lamb in a roasting tin and roast for 4–5 hours, until it is so tender you can prise the meat from the bone with a fork. Leave to rest for at least 20 minutes, up to an hour.

④ To prepare the cauliflower, warm some oil in a large sauté pan or frying pan and sauté the florets until golden brown all over; this should take 15–20 minutes. If your pan isn't large enough, you may need to do this in batches. Once all the cauliflower is browned, return all of it to the pan, pour in the vinegar and let bubble to reduce down to a glaze.

For the coconut and apple salad:
- ½ young coconut, skinned and thinly sliced
- 1 Granny Smith apple, cut into thin batons
- ½ small bunch of coriander (about 10g), leaves picked from stems
- ½ cucumber, halved lengthways, deseeded and sliced
- 1 red onion, halved and sliced
- 1 tbsp sesame oil
- Finely grated zest and juice of ½ lime

5 Add the cumin seeds and then pour in the coconut cream. Bring to the boil and let the liquor reduce until the cauliflower florets are nicely coated. Season with salt and pepper to taste and set aside.

6 For the salad, toss all the ingredients together in a bowl, season with salt and pepper and leave to stand for 10 minutes to allow the flavours to develop.

7 Carve the lamb and serve with the pan-fried cauliflower and coconut and apple salad.

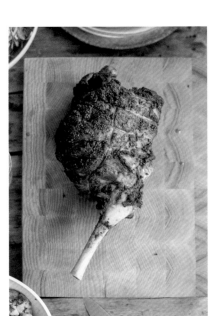

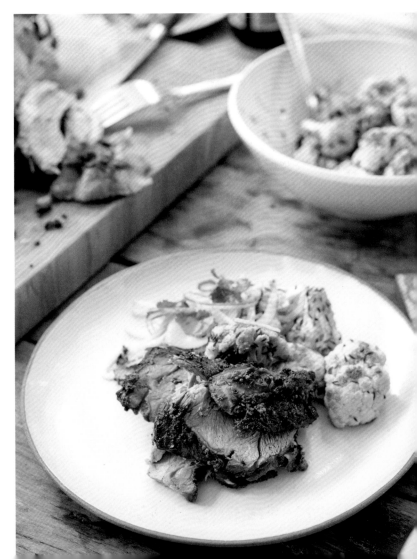

Rib eye steak chasseur

You've probably had the classic French chasseur sauce with game or poultry, but its rich flavour and robust texture work well with other meats too, and I think it goes fantastically with steak. The crumble topping lends that all-important crunch.

Serves: 4

Carb count: 8g per person

For the steaks:
Vegetable oil, for cooking
100g butter
4 rib eye steaks (about 250g each)
2 banana shallots, diced
1 chicken stock cube
1 tbsp tomato purée
75ml white wine vinegar
200g button mushrooms, sliced
200ml tinned beef consommé
    (I like Campbell's)
1 tsp cracked black pepper
Sea salt and freshly ground
    black pepper

For the crumble topping:
70g packet of pork scratchings,
    roughly crushed in the bag with
    a rolling pin
2 tbsp dried onion flakes
2 tsp thyme leaves
50g small bacon lardons, fried
    until crisp

1 Heat a large frying pan over a medium-high heat and add a little oil then 50g of the butter. Season the steaks with salt and pepper. Add them to the pan once the butter has stopped foaming and cook until well browned on both sides and to your liking. For medium-rare, allow 3–4 minutes on each side. Lift the steaks onto a warm plate to rest while you make the sauce.

2 Melt the remaining butter in the pan over a medium-low heat. When it stops foaming, add the shallots and sweat gently, stirring from time to time, for about 5 minutes until they are softened.

3 Crumble in the stock cube, stir in the tomato purée and cook, stirring, for 2–3 minutes. Add the wine vinegar and let bubble until reduced to a glaze. Stir in the mushrooms.

4 Pour in the beef consommé, increase the heat and simmer to reduce to a thick sauce, about 5 minutes. Season with the cracked pepper, and salt if you think it needs it. Stir in any juices that have accumulated on the steak plate.

5 For the crumble topping, in a small bowl, mix the pork scratchings with the onion flakes, thyme leaves and fried lardons.

6 Place the steaks on warm plates, spoon on the mushroom sauce then scatter over the crumble topping. Serve with a crisp green salad if you like.

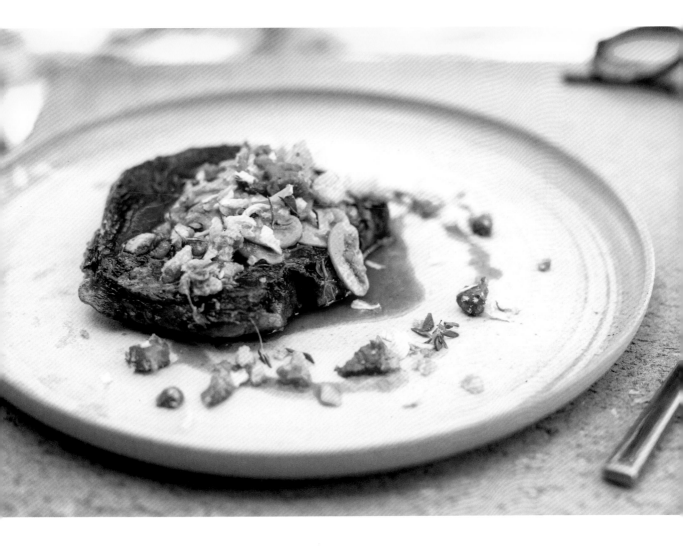

Barbecue-style brisket with red cabbage salad

I love this recipe because it means you can bring a bit of barbecue sunshine to the table even when it's raining! Of course, this tasty brisket is great cooked slowly in a covered barbecue, but the most consistent way to cook it is in the oven. The spice rub is good on chicken and pork too: double or triple up the quantities and keep the excess sealed in a jar in a cool, dark place, ready to add flavour to roasts whenever you like; it will keep for 2–3 months.

Serves: 6

Carb count: 16g per person

2kg beef brisket, in one piece

For the dry rub:
2 tbsp coriander seeds
2 tbsp cumin seeds
2 tbsp yellow mustard seeds
2 tbsp black peppercorns
2 tsp rock salt
2 tbsp smoked paprika
2 tsp cayenne pepper
1 tsp erythritol (sugar replacement)

For the red cabbage salad:
½ small red cabbage, cored and thinly sliced
1 white radish (also called mooli or daikon), peeled and cut into julienne
1 onion, halved and thinly sliced
2 tbsp flaky sea salt
100ml cider vinegar
2 tsp erythritol (sugar replacement)
100ml good-quality extra virgin olive oil
2 tbsp yellow mustard seeds, toasted in a dry frying pan until they start to pop
A bunch of dill (about 20g), fronds picked from stems

1 For the dry rub, put the coriander, cumin and mustard seeds, peppercorns and salt into a dry frying pan and toast over a medium heat until fragrant and starting to pop – be careful not to scorch them. Tip onto a plate to cool, then grind to a powder using a pestle and mortar. Mix with the smoked paprika, cayenne pepper and erythritol.

2 Score the brisket with a knife and massage the dry spice mix all over the meat and into the cuts. Wrap in cling film, place on a plate and leave to marinate in the fridge overnight.

3 Preheat the oven to 160°C/Fan 140°C/Gas 3. Place the brisket on a rack in a roasting tray and cover the tray tightly with foil. Roast in the oven for 5 hours.

4 For the salad, put the red cabbage, radish and onion into a bowl, sprinkle on the salt, mix well and leave to stand for 10 minutes.

5 In a small pan, heat the cider vinegar with the erythritol and simmer to reduce by half. Whisk in the olive oil and mustard seeds.

6 Tip the cabbage mix into a colander and wash off the salt under cold running water. Drain and pat dry on a clean tea towel.

For the barbecue sauce:
200ml beef stock
150ml red wine vinegar
100ml Diet Coke
75ml Sriracha sauce
50ml Worcestershire sauce
3 tbsp American-style mustard
3 tbsp tomato purée

⑦ Tip the cabbage into a bowl and pour on the vinegar mix. Stir, then cover and refrigerate.

⑧ Meanwhile, for the barbecue sauce, mix all of the ingredients together and set aside.

⑨ After 5 hours, take the brisket from the oven, remove the foil then pour on the barbecue sauce. Return to the oven for 1 hour, basting every 10 minutes, until the sauce forms a lovely glaze or crust on the beef. Remove from the oven and leave to rest for 20 minutes.

⑩ Just before serving, place the roasting tray over a medium heat and give the pan juices a good stir. Toss the dill through the cabbage. Serve the brisket with the pan juices spooned over and the red cabbage salad on the side.

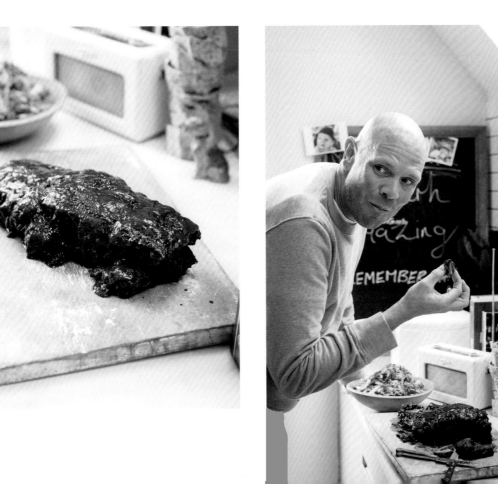

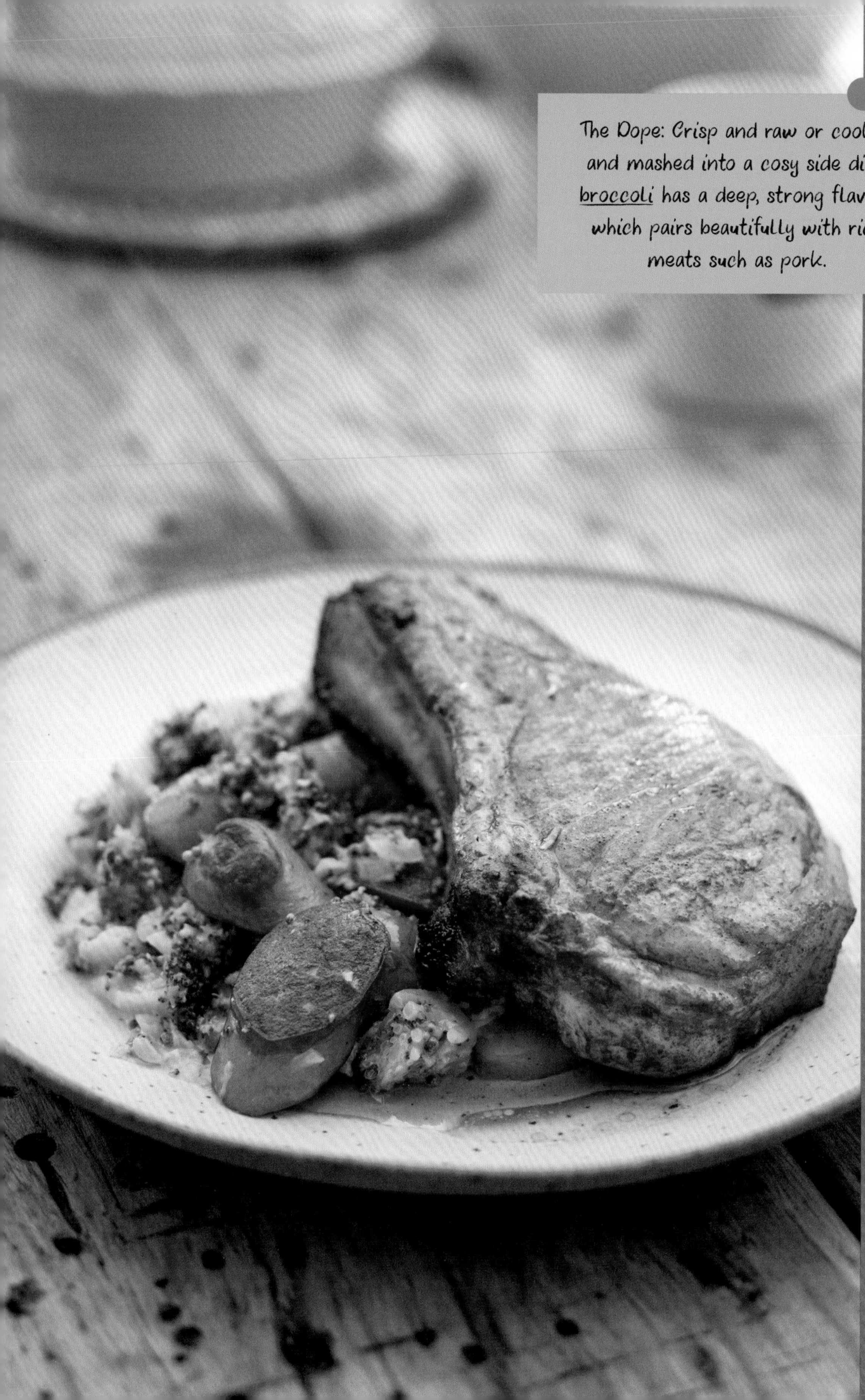

The Dope: Crisp and raw or cooked and mashed into a cosy side dish, broccoli has a deep, strong flavour which pairs beautifully with rich meats such as pork.

Pork chops with frankfurters and broccoli

This satisfying dinner takes everyday ingredients to a tasty new level. I usually try to keep veg nice and perky, but for this dish I cook the broccoli until it's quite soft (like mash) to complement the highly seasoned pork chops.

Serves: 2

Carb count: 22g per person

For the broccoli and frankfurters:
2 heads of broccoli (about 600g in total), cut into florets
50g butter
1 onion, diced
2 garlic cloves, grated
Vegetable oil, for cooking
2 best-quality jumbo frankfurters (about 200g in total), cut into 4cm slices
1 chicken stock cube
2 tbsp crème fraîche
2 tbsp yellow mustard seeds, toasted in a dry frying pan until they start to pop
4 pickled green chillies, finely chopped

For the pork chops:
2 large pork chops
2 tsp smoked paprika
Vegetable oil, for cooking
25g butter
Juice of 1 lemon
Sea salt and freshly ground black pepper

1 Bring a large pan of salted water to the boil, add the broccoli and simmer until just cooked, about 4–5 minutes. Drain in a colander, pat dry with kitchen paper and roughly chop; set aside.

2 Season the pork chops with salt and pepper then rub the smoked paprika all over them. Warm a large frying pan over a medium heat, add a splash of oil, then place the chops in the pan. Cook for about 4 minutes on each side, until well coloured and crisp. Add the butter and then the lemon juice. Baste the chops over the heat for 2–3 minutes, then transfer them to a warmed plate to rest.

3 While the chops are frying, warm the butter for the broccoli in a saucepan over a medium-low heat and sweat the onion and garlic, stirring from time to time, for 10–15 minutes until soft.

4 In a separate non-stick frying pan, warm a large splash of oil and fry the frankfurter slices until crisp and brown. Remove and drain on kitchen paper.

5 Add the cooked broccoli to the sautéed onion. Crumble in the stock cube, pour in 200ml water and bring to the boil. Simmer to reduce to a glaze. Stir in the crème fraîche, mustard seeds and fried frankfurters, then the pickled chillies. Season with salt and pepper to taste. Serve on warmed plates, with the pork chops.

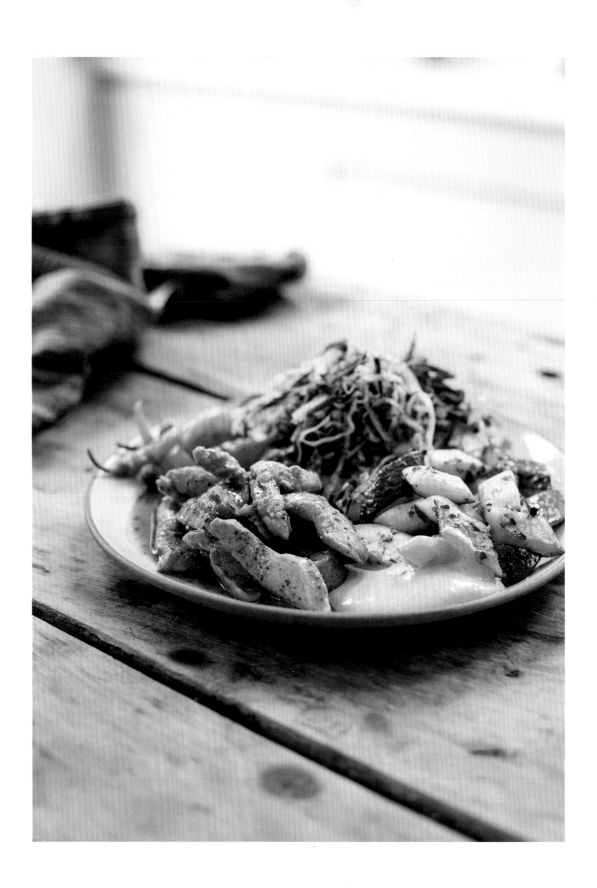

Hot pork strips with kebab dressing

This has everything you really want from a kebab: heat, crunch, fragrant pork and colourful veg, so it appeals to all the senses. There is just no pitta bread, but there's so much going on you're not going to miss it.

Serves: 4

Carb count: 21g per person

900g pork fillet, trimmed
75ml good-quality extra virgin olive oil
Finely grated zest and juice of 1 lemon
2 tbsp white wine vinegar
3 garlic cloves, grated
1 tsp ground cumin
1 tsp dried oregano
1 tsp dried thyme
1 tsp sea salt
1 tsp cracked black pepper
Vegetable oil, for frying
200ml chicken gravy (I make it with Bisto gravy granules)

For the salads:
¼ white cabbage, cored and thinly sliced
¼ red cabbage, cored and thinly sliced
1 onion, halved and thinly sliced
½ bunch of coriander (about 15g), roughly chopped, tender stems and all
½ bunch of mint (about 15g), tough stems removed, leaves roughly chopped
4 courgettes, halved lengthways, deseeded and cut into chunks
½ tsp dried chilli flakes, or to taste
90g thick mayonnaise
2 tsp Sriracha sauce
20 pickled green chillies, or more
Flaky sea salt

1 Cut the pork into 5cm strips. In a large bowl, whisk together the olive oil, lemon zest and juice, wine vinegar, garlic, cumin, oregano, thyme, salt and pepper. Add the pork, turn to coat and leave to marinate for 20 minutes.

2 Put all the cabbage into a large bowl, add the onion and sprinkle with 1 tbsp flaky salt. Mix with your hands then set aside for 10 minutes until softened. Tip into a colander, rinse under cold running water and pat dry with a clean tea towel or kitchen paper. Place in a bowl and toss with the coriander and mint. Keep to one side.

3 Heat a large frying pan over a high heat and add a little oil. Lift the pork out of the marinade with a slotted spoon and add to the pan. Fry the strips until just cooked; this should take only 4–5 minutes. Pour in the gravy and stir until it is hot and the pork is well coated.

4 While the pork is cooking, heat a splash of oil in another frying pan over a medium-high heat, add the courgettes and fry until just softened, about 5 minutes. Season with flaky sea salt and the chilli flakes. In a bowl, mix the mayonnaise and Sriracha sauce together to make a thick, spicy dressing.

5 Serve the pork, salads, spicy dressing and pickled chillies together in the middle of the table, so everyone can help themselves.

Roast shoulder of pork with rhubarb

You can't beat slow-roasted pork as a crowd pleaser, and here I've teamed it with rhubarb, which not only looks gorgeous, but it has an acidity that cuts through the richness of the meat beautifully.

Serves: 6

Carb count: 15g per person

1 shoulder of pork (about 3.5kg), bone in

For the brine:
500g rock salt
100ml dark soy sauce
50g knob of fresh ginger, thinly sliced
5 star anise
3 dried chillies

For the pickled rhubarb:
100ml cider vinegar
3 tbsp clear honey
1 tbsp erythritol (sugar replacement)
8 thin sticks of rhubarb, trimmed and cut into 10cm lengths

For the rhubarb purée:
200g butter
60g erythritol (sugar replacement)
600g rhubarb, chopped

1 First, make the brine. Pour 6 litres cold water into a large saucepan and add the salt, soy sauce, ginger, star anise and dried chillies. Bring to the boil, stirring occasionally to help dissolve the salt. Take off the heat and leave to cool.

2 Place the pork in a large container and pour on the cooled brine, including the aromatics. Cover with a lid or cling film and leave in the fridge for 6–8 hours.

3 Preheat the oven to 140°C/Fan 120°C/Gas 1. Lift the shoulder of pork from the brine and place it in a roasting tin. Roast for 4–5 hours, until the meat is very tender and can be shredded with a fork.

4 While the pork is in the oven, prepare the rhubarb. For the pickled rhubarb, pour 100ml water into a saucepan and add the cider vinegar, honey and erythritol. Bring to the boil and simmer for a couple of minutes. Lower the heat, add the rhubarb and simmer very gently for 3–5 minutes. Remove and leave the rhubarb to cool in the liquor. (You can prepare this up to a week ahead and keep it in a large, sterilised jar in the fridge until ready to serve.)

5 To make the rhubarb purée, warm the butter and erythritol in a heavy-bottomed saucepan over a medium heat. When the butter stops foaming, add the rhubarb and sweat gently until very soft, about 8–10 minutes. Pour into a jug blender and blitz to a smooth purée. (You can also do this with a stick blender.) Pass through a fine sieve and keep warm.

 Once cooked, let the pork rest for 20 minutes. Pull the meat into flakes with a fork and serve with the pickled rhubarb and rhubarb purée.

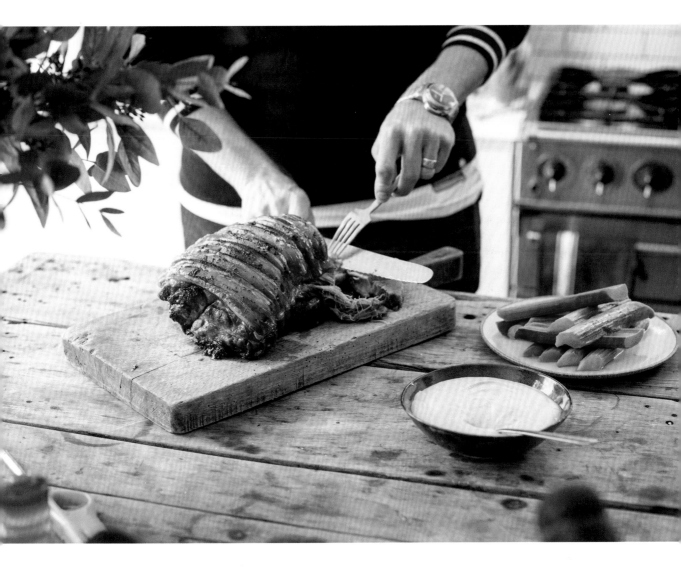

Gammon with cabbage wedges and apples

This one-pan wonder is just the thing for an easy weeknight dinner. It might not be the prettiest dish, but it's definitely one of the tastiest. Use the best frankfurters you can find, with a high meat content – it will make all the difference.

Serves: 2
Carb count: 27g per person

75g butter
2 onions, halved and thinly sliced
2 garlic cloves, sliced
1 medium Savoy cabbage, trimmed
4 best-quality frankfurters
2 Granny Smith apples, peeled,
    cored and quartered
400ml chicken stock
3 tbsp yellow mustard seeds,
    toasted in a dry frying pan just
    until they begin to pop
2 tbsp Dijon mustard
2 large, thick gammon steaks
    (about 250g each)
Sea salt and freshly ground
    black pepper

1 Preheat the oven to 180°C/Fan 160°C/Gas 4. Place a roasting tin on the hob over a medium heat and add the butter. Once melted, add the onions and garlic and sweat, stirring from time to time, for about 10 minutes until soft.

2 Cut the Savoy cabbage into quarters (or into 6 wedges if it is a bit larger), keeping the root intact so each holds together. Place the cabbage wedges on top of the onions, then add the frankfurters and apples. Pour on the stock and stir in the mustard seeds and Dijon mustard.

3 Lay the gammon steaks on top and bring to the boil. Cover the tray tightly with foil and cook in the oven for 30–35 minutes. Take out of the oven and carefully lift off the foil. Remove the gammon and frankfurters to a warmed plate.

4 Place the roasting tray back on the hob and let bubble to reduce the sauce until thickened to a nice gravy. Season with salt and pepper to taste.

5 Halve the frankfurters and cut each gammon steak into 2 or 3 pieces. Divide the cabbage between warmed plates, top with the meat and pour on the sauce. Serve straight away.

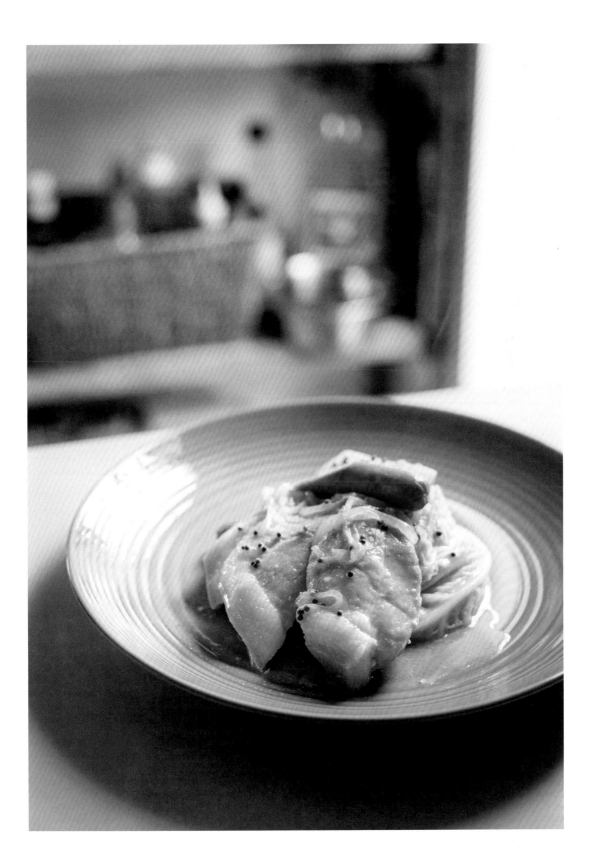

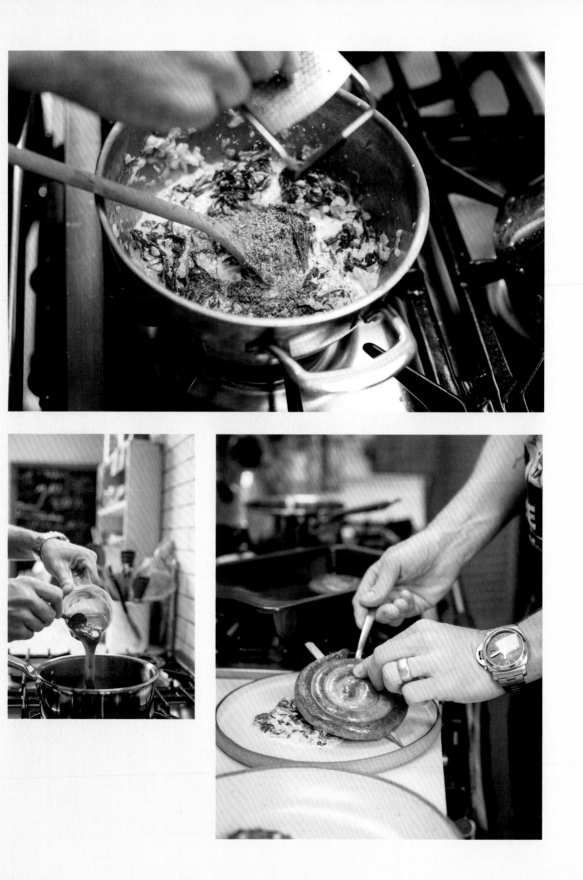

Cumberland sausages with onion gravy

Sausages with onion gravy is a pub classic and family favourite that we would typically serve with piles of mashed potato. Here, I've replaced the usual high-carb mash with comforting creamed spinach, so you don't miss the mash at all.

Serves: 2

Carb count: 38g per person

Vegetable oil, for cooking
2 large Cumberland sausage rings

For the onion gravy:
1 onion, halved and thinly sliced
100ml balsamic vinegar
200ml chicken stock
150ml chicken gravy (I make it
 with Bisto gravy granules)
1 tbsp English mustard
1 tbsp wholegrain mustard

For the creamed spinach:
400g baby spinach
40g butter
1 onion, diced
2 garlic cloves, grated
250ml double cream
¼–½ tsp freshly grated nutmeg
Sea salt and freshly ground
 black pepper

1 Preheat the oven to 180°C/Fan 160°C/Gas 4. Heat a large non-stick frying pan over a medium heat and add a splash of oil. Sear the sausage rings, one at a time, on both sides then transfer them to a roasting tin. Roast in the oven for 15–20 minutes, until cooked through.

2 While the sausages are cooking, for the gravy, warm a splash of oil in a pan over a medium-low heat and gently sweat the onion, stirring occasionally, for 10–15 minutes until softened.

3 Meanwhile, put the spinach into a colander in the sink and pour on boiling water from the kettle to wilt it. Use a clean tea towel or kitchen paper to squeeze out excess water.

4 Heat the butter in a saucepan over a medium-low heat. Add the onion and garlic and sweat gently, stirring occasionally, for 10–15 minutes until softened. Pour in the cream and simmer to reduce by half. Stir in the wilted spinach and cook gently for 2–3 minutes. Season with the nutmeg, and salt and pepper to taste.

5 To make the gravy, add the balsamic vinegar to the softened onion, increase the heat a bit and reduce to a glaze. Pour on the stock and reduce by half, then add the chicken gravy and bring to the boil. Whisk in the mustards.

6 Serve the sausages with loads of gravy and the creamed spinach on the side.

Gammon steaks with fried duck eggs

Served with a hot gherkin gravy, this is a smartened up version of the ham-and-egg teas of my childhood. You have to be a bit fast and furious to get it all ready at the same time, but it's not difficult as long as you have all the ingredients prepared before you start. Serve it simply, with some lightly cooked greens or a nice, crunchy slaw (see pages 130 and 168). And be sure to ask your butcher for the best gammon steaks they have.

Serves: 4

Carb count: 9g per person

4 thick gammon steaks
Vegetable oil, for cooking
4 duck eggs
¼ tsp dried chilli flakes
Sea salt and freshly ground
  black pepper

For the hot gherkin gravy:
100g pancetta, diced
1 onion, finely diced
1 garlic clove, grated
½ tsp chilli powder
¼ tsp cayenne pepper
¼ tsp smoked paprika
2 large dill pickles, sliced into
  discs, plus 50ml pickle liquor
  from the jar
250ml chicken gravy (I make it
  with Bisto gravy granules)
60g pork scratchings, lightly
  crushed

To finish:
Dill fronds

1 First, start making the gherkin gravy. Place the pancetta in a small saucepan over a medium-high heat until it renders its fat and becomes crisp. Scoop it out with a slotted spoon and set aside. Add the onion to the pan and sweat gently, stirring from time to time, for about 10 minutes until soft.

2 While the onion is cooking, preheat the grill to hot. Grill the gammon steaks for 3–4 minutes each side; keep warm.

3 Once the onion is softened, add the garlic to the pan and cook, stirring, for a minute. Sprinkle in the chilli powder, cayenne and smoked paprika and cook for 2–3 minutes. Add the dill pickle liquor and chicken gravy and bring to the boil. Stir in the reserved pancetta, sliced pickles and pork scratchings. Keep warm.

4 Heat a little oil in a non-stick frying pan and fry the duck eggs until the whites are set, and a little crispy at the edges if you like. Season with salt, pepper and the dried chilli flakes.

5 Place a gammon steak on each warmed plate and top with a fried egg. Spoon on the gravy and scatter over the dill. Serve immediately.

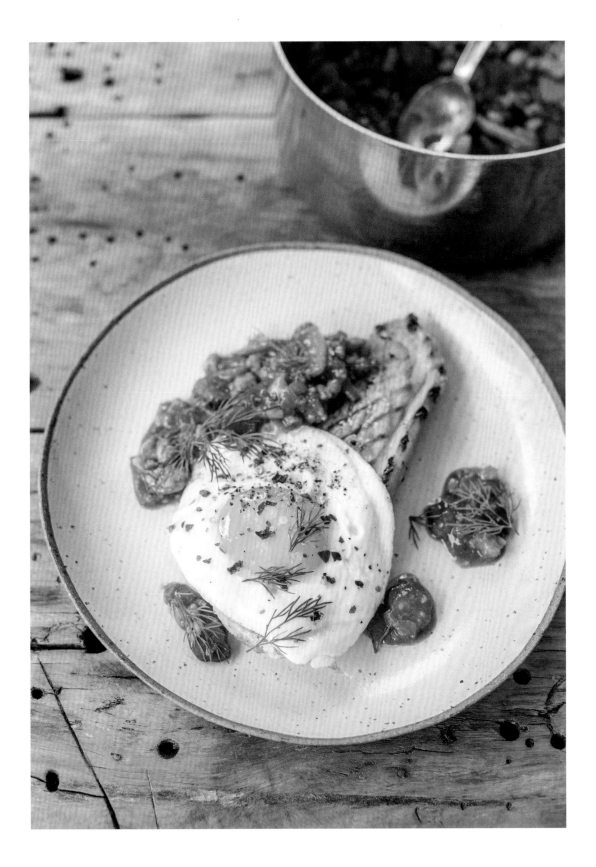

Indulgent and delicious

SWEET THINGS & BAKING

RECKON WE ARE MATES BY NOW so I can be honest and tell you that this chapter was the biggest challenge of all. Working out how to replace bread, crackers, biscuits, cakes and puddings while trying to stay low-carb is tough.

In some cases, it's a question of shifting your expectations because gluten-free bread is never going to have that lovely chewy tang of a great slice of sourdough. You need gluten for that and for gluten you need carb-heavy wheat flour. But you know what? If you just fancy a slice of toast, the almond soda bread (page 257) spread generously with butter or topped with cheese and grilled isn't half bad. And almonds are a really good source of phenylalanine, an amino acid that's essential for the production of dopamine.

The flaxseed biscuits (page 254) are so good, I would happily put them on the menu at The Hand and Flowers to go with cheese. Flaxseeds have a carb content, but it's a fibrous carbohydrate, making it a low-GI food that won't cause your blood sugar levels to spike after eating it.

When it comes to sweet things, I'm not going to lie. If you're out with your friends and someone is having a wonderful sticky toffee pudding with gorgeous vanilla ice cream and loads of toffee sauce, you'd be an idiot not to want that too. The thought that you can't have it can be a bit of a downer.

These are the times when you have to think about what you're gaining. It's in this chapter that I think you might really have the sense that you're making a big shift in how you eat, but I hope I've come up with some good ideas for what to do when you just want something sweet, or you are having friends round and you want a show-stopping pud that both tastes and looks delicious.

I've tried to create satisfying alternatives for the sort of desserts we all crave from time to time. The crème brûlée (page 242) has the same sort of creamy cosiness that you get from a traditional one and, though I say so myself, the tiramisu (page 245) is exceptionally good. The strawberry cheesecake (page 246) is a brilliant crowd pleaser too. No one will ever guess these puds don't have conventional sugars in them, I promise.

I have to say a word here about the sugar replacements I've used in this book, because some of you might be surprised that a chef like me would consider such things. It all goes along with having to make a big change to get a big change. A bit like with booze (see page 18), having a little sugar can quickly turn into having a lot, and then you're right back where you started.

In the recipes here, I use both erythritol and inulin to replace conventional sugar. These are called 'sugar alcohols' – though they're not alcohol and they're not sugar – and they don't affect blood sugar levels in the way that ordinary sugars do. Used as part of a low-carbohydrate diet, they work very well to help you deal with those moments or occasions when only something sweet will do.

Quick treats

Sometimes, when I feel like I want to accelerate my weight loss, I give up sugar entirely. I often think it's easier not to yield to temptation at all, to cut it out completely. But then again, I'm in this for the long haul, so when I'm really craving something sweet, this is what I reach for:

* A square or two of really good-quality dark chocolate, at least 70 per cent cocoa solids
* A handful of grapes, ideally really cold from the fridge
* A small bowl of ripe, flavourful tyrosine-rich strawberries or blueberries
* A small piece of the coffee and walnut cake used in the tiramisu (page 245)
* Slices of apple spread with a bit of peanut butter. Note that apples contain the antioxidant quercetin, which may help the brain prevent dopamine loss.

Blueberry bread and butter pudding

This is just the thing when you're craving a little something sweet. I find inulin (a polysaccharide which is mildly sweet and often extracted from chicory root) caramelises the pudding quite well and gives a lovely finish; it is available online.

Serves: 4–6

Carb count: 10–7g per person

About 140g butter, softened,
   for greasing and spreading
1 almond soda bread loaf
   (page 257), thinly sliced
½ tsp freshly grated nutmeg
600ml double cream
2 vanilla pods, split lengthways,
   seeds scraped out
8 large free-range egg yolks
20g erythritol (sugar replacement)
100g blueberries
1–2 tbsp inulin (sugar replacement,
   see page 242), to glaze

① Lightly butter an ovenproof serving dish, about 23cm square and 5cm deep. Butter each slice of bread and lay the slices on a large board then sprinkle evenly with the nutmeg.

② Pour the cream into a saucepan, add the vanilla seeds and pods and heat slowly until bubbles form at the edge. Meanwhile, whisk the egg yolks and erythritol together in a bowl.

③ Pour the hot cream onto the egg mixture, whisking all of the time, then pour back into the rinsed-out saucepan. Cook, stirring, over a medium heat until the custard thickens slightly, about 4–5 minutes. Pass through a sieve into a jug.

④ Pour some custard into the prepared dish and sprinkle in a few blueberries. Cover with a layer of bread, buttered side up. Repeat to use up all of the ingredients, finishing with a layer of bread. Leave to stand for 25–30 minutes, to allow the bread to soak up the custard.

⑤ Preheat the oven to 130°C/Fan 110°/Gas ¾. Stand the dish on a baking sheet and bake for 25–30 minutes, until the custard has just set. Remove and leave to stand for 10 minutes.

⑥ Sprinkle the inulin over the top of the pudding and glaze with a cook's blowtorch (or briefly under a preheated very hot grill) until caramelised, then serve.

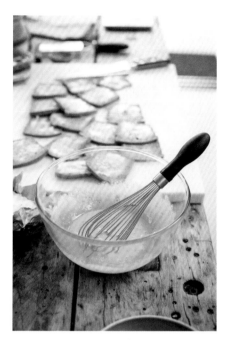

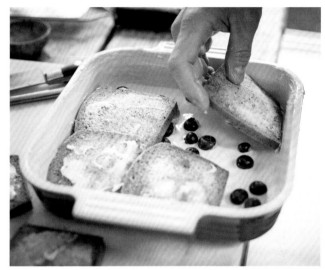

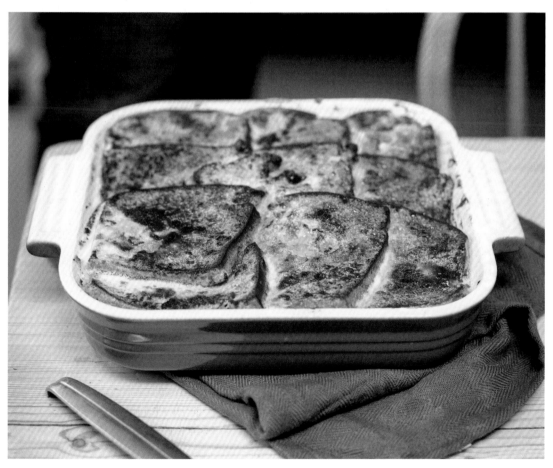

Crème brûlée

Simple, classic and very low in carbs, this is one of my all-time favourite desserts. In fact, this recipe is a version of the one we serve at The Hand and Flowers, adapted to use the sugar replacements I've found so useful. You can easily find erythritol and inulin online. Inulin is the only sugar substitute I've found that caramelises and sets like sugar, making it perfect for this classic dessert.

Serves: 6

Carb count: 3g per person

750ml double cream
2 vanilla pods, split lengthways
4 large free-range eggs
20g erythritol (sugar replacement)
6 tbsp inulin (sugar replacement),
   to glaze

1 Put the cream and vanilla pods into a heavy-bottomed saucepan and bring just to the boil. Take the pan off the heat and leave to stand for 30 minutes.

2 Bring the infused cream back up to a simmer. Meanwhile, in a bowl, whisk the eggs and erythritol together to combine. Pour on the hot vanilla cream, whisking as you do so, then pour the vanilla custard back into the rinsed-out saucepan.

3 Cook the custard, stirring constantly with a wooden spoon, over a medium-low heat until it thickens enough to lightly coat the back of the spoon; it should register 87°C on a cook's thermometer.

4 Pass the custard through a fine sieve into a bowl and leave to cool for 20 minutes.

5 Once cooled, scrape the custard into a blender and blitz for 20 seconds – this will give it a nice, glossy finish.

6 Divide the mixture between 6 ramekins or similar heatproof serving dishes. Refrigerate for at least 4 hours, or overnight, to set.

When you're ready to serve, sprinkle the inulin on top of the set custards in a nice, even layer. Using a cook's blowtorch, **7** caramelise the inulin until it forms a deep, caramel crust (or place briefly under a preheated very hot grill). Leave for a minute or so to allow the glaze to set before serving.

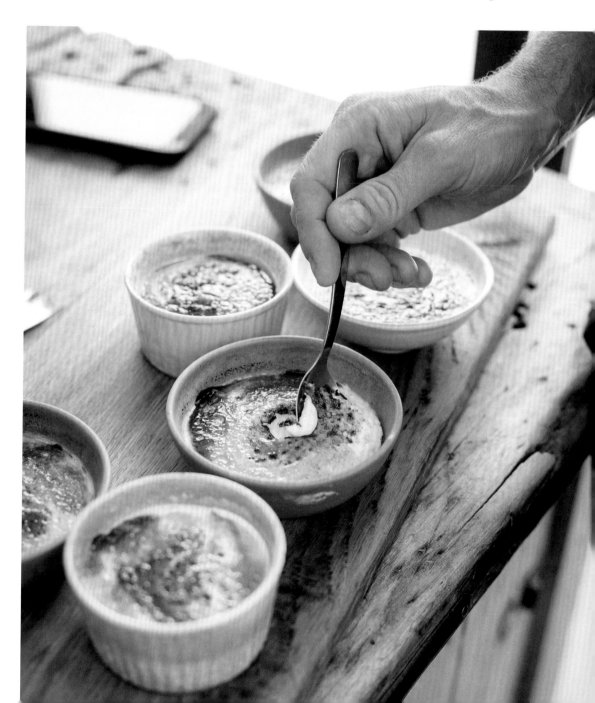

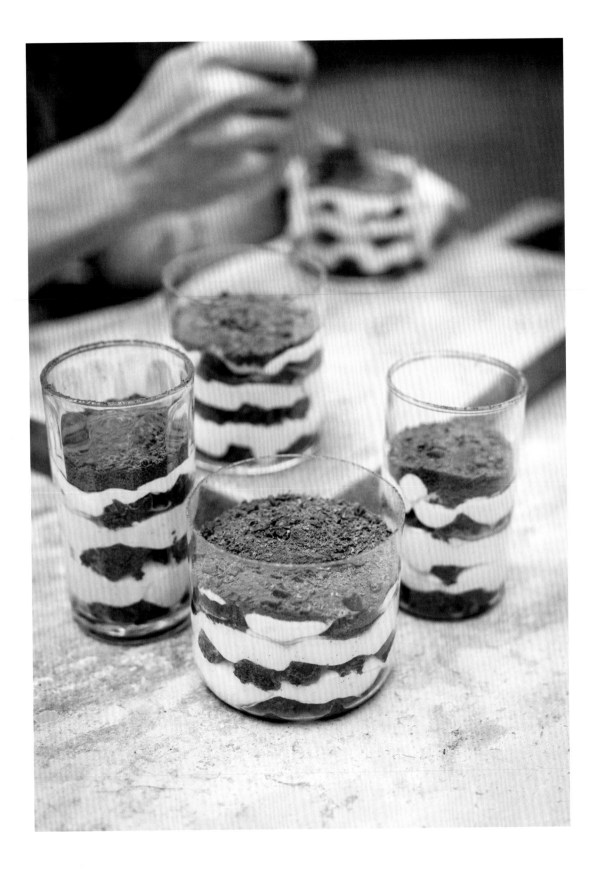

Tiramisu

I'm not embarrassed to say that this is an amazing version of that classic Italian dessert. I promise you, it's as good as one that's loaded with carbs. If you don't have an espresso machine, just get some from your favourite coffee shop or use a good instant espresso powder.

Serves: 6
Carb count: 10g per person

For the coffee and walnut cake:
150g vegetable oil, plus extra
    for oiling
100g ground almonds
90g ground flaxseed
50g erythritol (sugar replacement)
7g good-quality instant coffee
    (I use Nescafé Azera Intenso)
1 tsp bicarbonate of soda
50g walnut oil
150g grated Granny Smith apple
4 large free-range eggs, lightly
    beaten

For the mascarpone cream:
400ml double cream
260g mascarpone
60g erythritol (sugar replacement)
2 large vanilla pods, split
    lengthways, seeds scraped out

For the coffee:
6 espressos (see above), or strong
    coffee made with good instant
    coffee (warm or cold is fine)

For the topping:
2 tbsp cocoa powder
2 tbsp roughly crushed coffee
    beans
50g dark chocolate (80 per cent
    cocoa solids)

❶ Preheat the oven to 120°C/Fan 100°C/Gas ½. Lightly oil a 450g loaf tin or 20cm springform cake tin, then line with baking parchment and oil the parchment.

❷ To make the cake, put all of the ingredients into the bowl of a stand mixer fitted with the paddle attachment and beat on a medium-low speed until it forms a light batter. Pour into the prepared tin and bake for 1 hour, until a wooden skewer inserted into the middle of the cake comes out clean. Leave to cool in the tin for 10 minutes, then transfer it to a wire rack to cool completely.

❸ For the mascarpone cream, place the cream, mascarpone, erythritol and vanilla seeds in a bowl and beat until smooth.

❹ Cut the cake into 1cm slices and arrange a layer in each of 6 serving glasses. Spoon about 1 tbsp espresso over each, then cover with a layer of mascarpone cream. Repeat these layers (cake, coffee, cream) three more times, ending with a cream layer.

❺ Sprinkle over the cocoa powder and coffee beans, then grate the chocolate all over the top. Chill for at least 3 hours, up to 2 days.

❻ Take the glasses of tiramisu out of the fridge about 20 minutes before serving.

Strawberry cheesecake

This cheesecake is so good that when it was first made and trialled for a staff tea at The Hand and Flowers, not a single person thought it was low-carb. It takes a bit of effort to knock up, but it's really worth it, particularly for a special meal.

Serves: 6–8

Carb count: 10–8g per person

For the base:
110g unsalted butter, melted, plus extra to grease the tin
100g ground almonds, lightly toasted in a dry frying pan until light golden
100g ground flaxseed
12g erythritol (sugar replacement)
1 tsp flaky sea salt

For the cheesecake layer:
500g strawberries
350g cream cheese, at room temperature
125g erythritol (sugar replacement)
6 sheets of leaf gelatine
280ml double cream
150g free-range egg whites (about 4 eggs)
4 free-range egg yolks
2 vanilla pods, split lengthways, seeds scraped out

To serve (optional):
Blueberries and halved strawberries

1 Lightly butter a deep, 20cm springform cake tin and line with baking parchment.

2 To make the base, put the ground almonds, flaxseed, erythritol and salt into a large bowl and stir with a wooden spoon until well mixed. Add the melted butter and mix to combine. Press the crumb-like mix evenly over the base of the prepared tin, right into the edges. Refrigerate to set for about an hour.

3 For the cheesecake, blitz the strawberries in a food processor then pass through a fine sieve; you need 300g purée. Using a stand mixer, or electric hand whisk and bowl, on a low speed, beat the cream cheese with the strawberry purée and 80g of the erythritol for a minute or so to combine. Scrape into a container. Wash and dry the bowl well.

4 Soak the gelatine in cold water to cover for 5 minutes. Whip the cream in a large bowl to soft peaks; set aside. Whisk the egg whites with 30g of the remaining erythritol in the cleaned mixer bowl to firm peaks; set aside.

5 Put the egg yolks, remaining 15g erythritol and vanilla seeds into a heatproof bowl over a pan of barely simmering water, making sure the bottom of the bowl does not touch the water. Whisk for about 5 minutes to a rich, thick sabayon; do not overheat or the eggs will scramble. Remove the bowl from the pan.

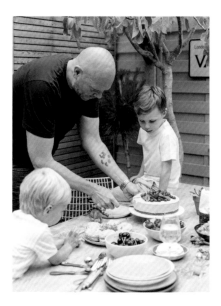

6 Drain the gelatine, squeeze out excess water and put into a small pan with 2 tbsp water. Warm over a very low heat just until it melts, then carefully fold into the warm sabayon.

7 The elements need to be combined lightly but thoroughly, keeping the mixture as light as possible. Fold the sabayon into the whipped cream, then fold this into the strawberry cream cheese. Finally, fold in the meringue, half at a time. Pour the mixture onto the base in the tin, cover and refrigerate overnight. Serve as it is or topped with fresh berries.

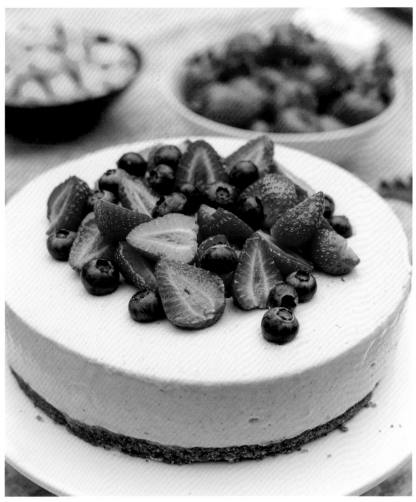

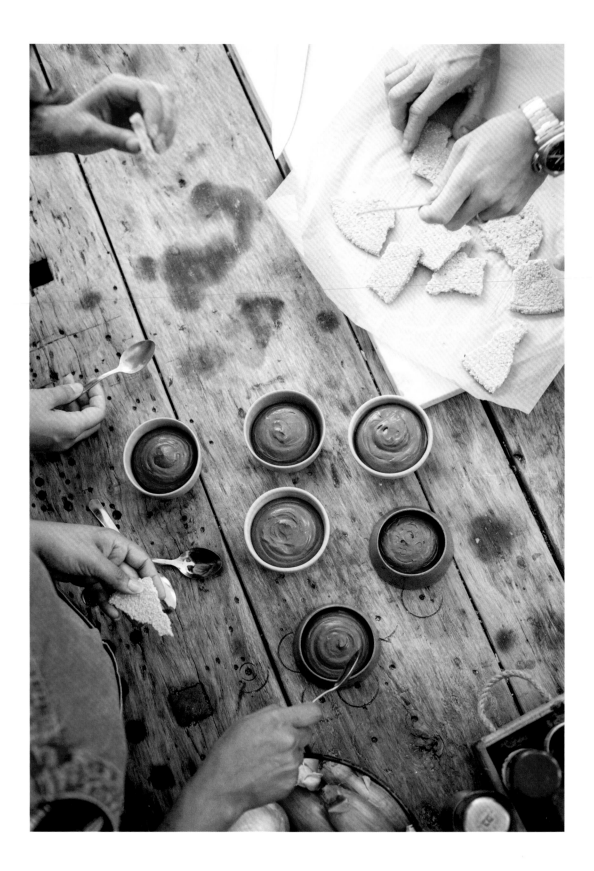

Chocolate mousse with sesame almond biscuits

This is the ideal quick and easy recipe to turn to when the craving for chocolate strikes. It's very low-carb yet really rich and tasty. The sesame almond biscuits are a lovely crisp contrast, and they make a nice little treat with a cup of tea too.

Serves: 6

Carb count: 8g per person

For the chocolate mousse:
600g cream cheese
90g cocoa powder
50g erythritol (sugar replacement)
2 vanilla pods, split lengthways,
    seeds scraped out
A pinch of salt
60g crème fraîche, beaten
    until soft

For the biscuits:
2 large free-range egg whites
1 tsp erythritol (sugar replacement)
100g ground almonds
50g sesame seeds
A pinch of salt

1 Using a stand mixer or electric hand whisk and bowl, beat the cream cheese, cocoa, erythritol, vanilla seeds and salt together until light, then fold in the crème fraîche.

2 Use a spatula to scrape the mixture into a piping bag fitted with a plain nozzle (or into a strong plastic bag and snip off the corner). Pipe the mousse into 6 ramekins or other individual dishes. Refrigerate for an hour or so to set.

3 Meanwhile, make the biscuits. Preheat the oven to 170°C/Fan 150°C/Gas 3½ and have ready a large baking sheet.

4 In a clean bowl, whisk the egg whites with the erythritol to soft peaks, then fold in the ground almonds, sesame seeds and salt to form a mixture that resembles pastry.

5 Roll out the mixture between 2 sheets of baking parchment to about the thickness of a £1 coin. Remove the top parchment, then lift onto the prepared baking sheet. Bake for 25–30 minutes until golden and crisp. Transfer to a wire rack and leave to cool.

6 Just before serving, break the sesame almond biscuit sheet up into pieces to serve alongside the chocolate mousse.

Coffee, chocolate and chia seed pudding

This is a very quick pudding – just mix it up and chill it in the fridge. The chia seeds make everything set to a soft, mousse-like texture. The pairing of orange and chocolate is always a winner and the coffee takes it to another level.

Serves: 4

Carb count: 14g per person

For the pudding:
500g wholemilk yoghurt
70g chia seeds
1 tbsp orange extract
2 tbsp cocoa powder
20ml freshly made espresso
1 tbsp erythritol (sugar
 replacement)

To finish:
About 2 tsp grated dark chocolate
 (80 per cent cocoa solids)
About 2 tsp cacao nibs
About 2 tsp roughly crushed
 espresso beans

1 Put the yoghurt into a bowl and whisk in the chia seeds, orange extract, cocoa powder, espresso and erythritol.

2 Spoon the mixture into 4 serving glasses, dividing it equally, and cover with cling film. Leave in the fridge for 12–24 hours.

3 When you're ready to serve, remove the puddings from the fridge and sprinkle evenly with the grated chocolate, cacao nibs and crushed espresso beans.

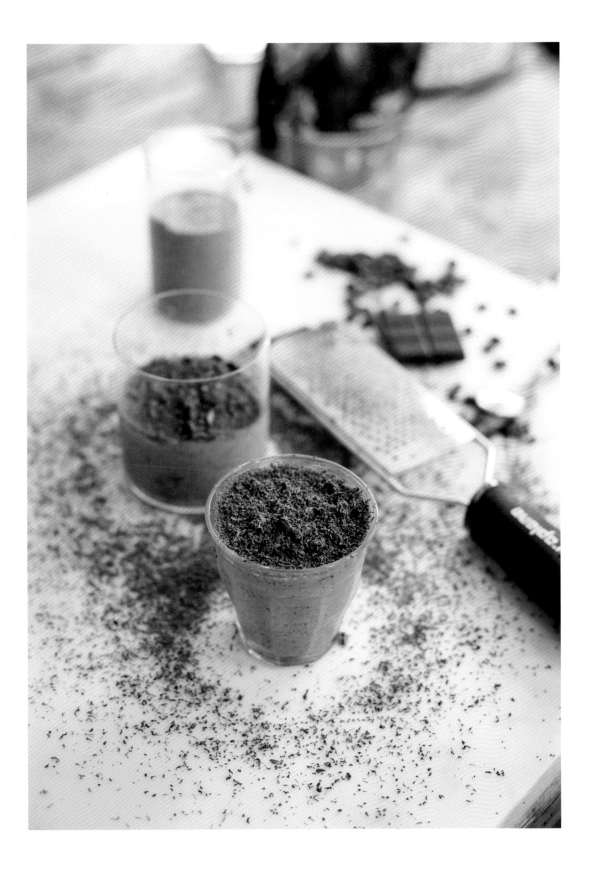

Sweet coconut and lavender 'puff burgers'

On the day we were photographing these, my mate Joel from the band The Rifles came over with his wife Gemma and their kids to help us eat all the food. We were wondering what to call these – they're not quite a meringue, not quite a macaron – and Joel came up with the name 'puff burgers', which was too good not to use!

Serves: 6
Carb count: 4g per person

For the coconut puffs:
140g free-range egg whites
   (about 4)
75g erythritol (sugar replacement)
½ tsp vanilla seeds (scraped out
   from about 2 large pods), or
   vanilla bean paste
¼ tsp cream of tartar
A pinch of salt
75g desiccated coconut, toasted
   until fragrant and golden in a
   dry frying pan

For the cream cheese filling:
100ml double cream
25g erythritol (sugar replacement)
75g cream cheese
1 tbsp culinary dried lavender
Finely grated zest of 1 lemon

To finish (optional):
60g dark chocolate (about
   70 per cent cocoa solids),
   in pieces

1 Preheat the oven to 110°C/Fan 90°C/Gas ¼. Line a couple of baking sheets with baking parchment. Draw six evenly spaced 7cm circles on each liner with a pencil and turn the paper over.

2 Using a stand mixer or electric hand whisk and bowl, whisk together the egg whites, erythritol, vanilla seeds (or paste), cream of tartar and salt until stiff peaks form. Using a large metal spoon or spatula, gently fold in the toasted coconut.

3 Spoon the mixture into a piping bag fitted with a plain nozzle and pipe twelve 7cm discs on the lined baking sheets, in the outlined circles. Bake for about 25 minutes, until the meringues take on a little colour. Turn the oven off and leave the meringues inside to dry out overnight.

4 When you're ready to assemble the coconut puffs, make the filling. In a bowl, whisk the cream with the erythritol until fairly stiff, but do not over-beat. In a separate bowl, beat the cream cheese, lavender and lemon zest together until smooth, then lightly fold in the whipped cream until evenly combined. Spoon the filling into a piping bag fitted with a large plain nozzle; set aside.

5 If finishing with chocolate, place it in a small heatproof bowl over a pan of barely simmering water – the bottom of the bowl shouldn't touch the water. Warm gently until melted and smooth then remove from the heat.

6 When you're ready to serve, pipe a generous amount of the cream cheese filling on the flat side of one of the coconut puffs, right to the edge. Top with another coconut puff, pressing it firmly against the cream to make sure it sits in place. Repeat with the rest of the meringue discs and filling. Lay the finished puffs on a wire rack and drizzle with melted chocolate to finish if you like.

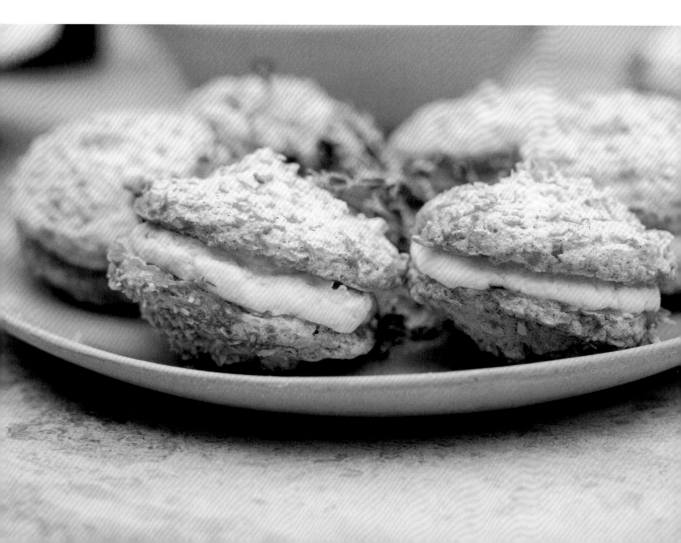

Flaxseed biscuits

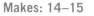

I am really pleased with these savoury biscuits – they don't taste low-carb at all! They are great with cheese or pâté, but they also work brilliantly crumbled on top of dishes that call for some added texture and crunch. They will keep in an airtight tin for up to a week.

Makes: 14–15	
Carb count: 1g per biscuit	

4 large free-range egg whites
20g erythritol (sugar replacement)
150g ground flaxseed
150g ground almonds
15g baking powder
A pinch of salt

1 Preheat the oven to 170°C/Fan 150°C/Gas 3. Line a couple of baking sheets with baking parchment.

2 Using a stand mixer, or electric hand whisk and bowl, whisk the egg whites and erythritol to stiff peaks. Fold in the ground flaxseed, ground almonds, baking powder and salt. Work until the dough is evenly combined and forms a ball.

3 Roll out the dough between two sheets of baking parchment to about a 5mm thickness. Remove the top sheet of parchment and cut out 7cm rounds from the dough. Gently re-roll any scraps and cut out more rounds.

4 Place the dough rounds on the prepared baking sheets and bake for 25–30 minutes.

5 Remove from the oven and leave the biscuits on the baking sheets for about 5 minutes to firm up, then transfer to a wire rack to cool.

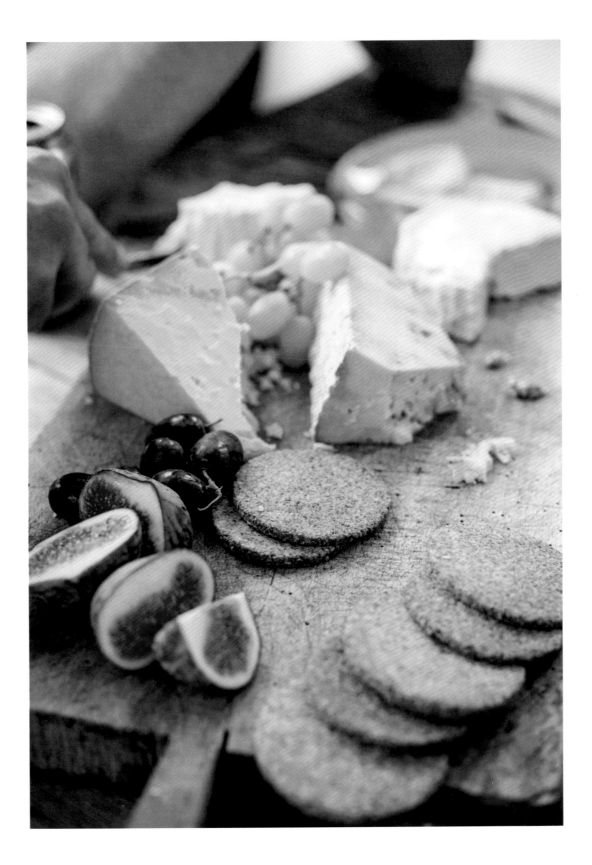

The Dope: Ground almonds add great texture and flavour to baking, providing an alternative to wheat flour. You can also use them to thicken sauces and to add a crunchy topping to casseroles and bakes.

Almond soda bread

I have to be honest, this isn't 'bread' as such. It's impossible to replicate a great sourdough loaf without wheat flour, but I think of this as a vehicle for other things – for those times when you want a quick snack or a simple breakfast or supper. Toasted and spread with loads of butter, it's pretty good!

Makes: 1 loaf, about 10 slices

Carb count: 2g per slice

60g butter, melted, plus extra
    to grease the tin
175g ground almonds
30g ground flaxseed
20g coconut flour
5 large free-range eggs, lightly
    beaten
1½ tbsp erythritol (sugar
    replacement)
1 tbsp white wine vinegar
1½ tsp salt
1½ tsp bicarbonate of soda

1 Preheat the oven to 180°C/Fan 160°C/Gas 4. Butter a 450g loaf tin, line it with baking parchment and butter the parchment.

2 Put all of the ingredients into a food processor and blend for 1 minute until well combined.

3 Tip the mixture into the prepared loaf tin and bake for 35 minutes until cooked through.

4 Leave the loaf in the tin on a wire rack for 10 minutes, then remove and place directly on the rack to cool completely before slicing.

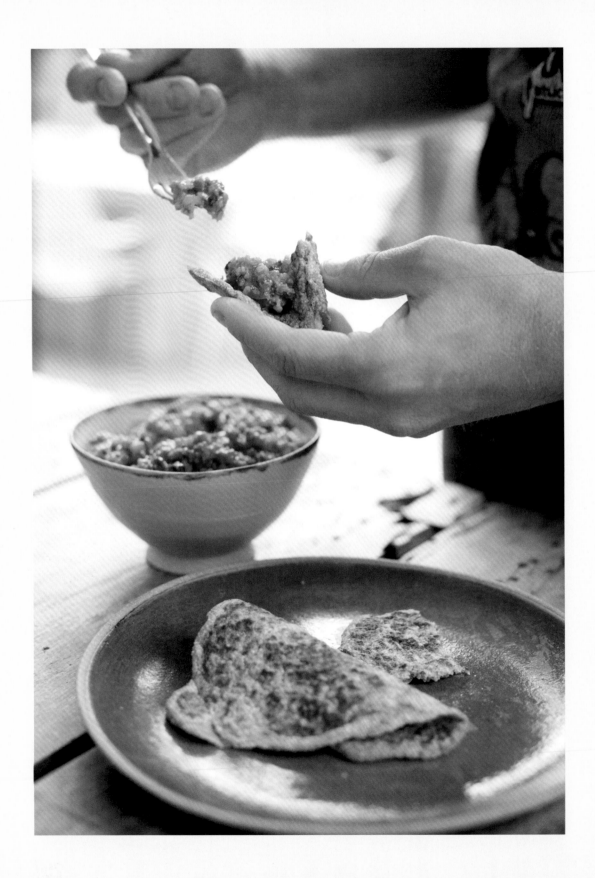

Flatbreads

I created these small flatbreads when I was trying to find a replacement for pitta and naan to go with the curries and spicy foods I love so much. They are best eaten very fresh and warm, so make them at the last minute and serve straight from the pan – with soups, curries and casseroles.

Makes: 6
Carb count: 3g per flatbread

40g butter
60g coconut flour
15g powdered psyllium husk
1 tsp baking powder
½ tsp salt

① Melt the butter in a small saucepan over a medium heat and cook until it is a nut brown colour and fragrant. Remove from the heat.

② In a bowl, whisk the coconut flour, psyllium husk, baking powder and salt together until well combined. Trickle on the brown butter and mix to a buttery paste.

③ Slowly pour on 250ml boiling water, stirring the mixture constantly with a spoon as you do so. Keep stirring until you end up with a smooth, stretchy dough.

④ Divide the dough into 6 small balls. One at a time, roll them out thinly between two sheets of baking parchment.

⑤ Heat a large, non-stick frying pan over a high heat. Cook the flatbreads, one at a time, for about a minute on each side. The dough will rise and become a light and toasty flatbread. Serve immediately.

Index

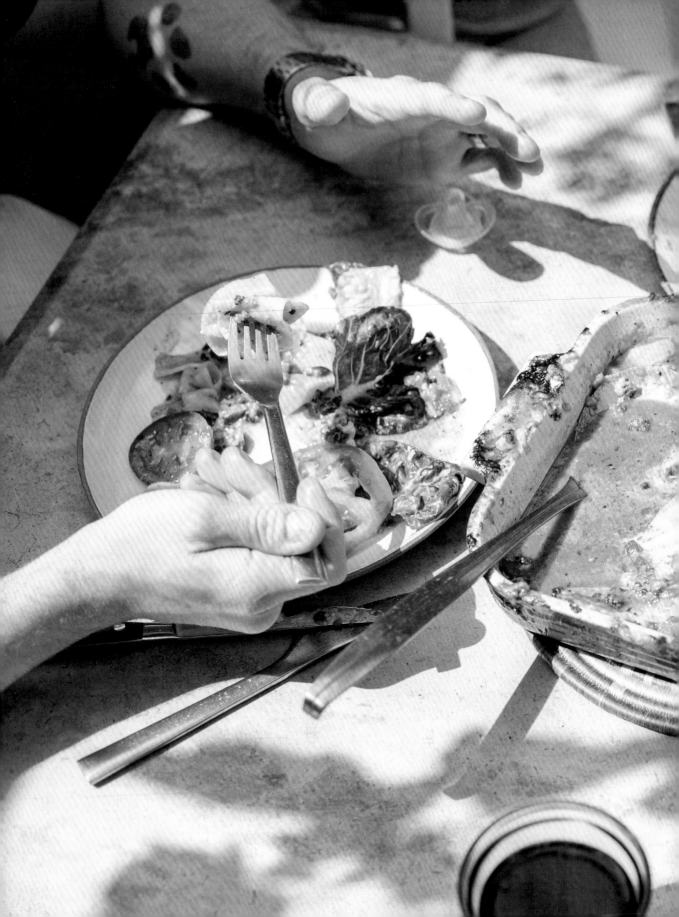

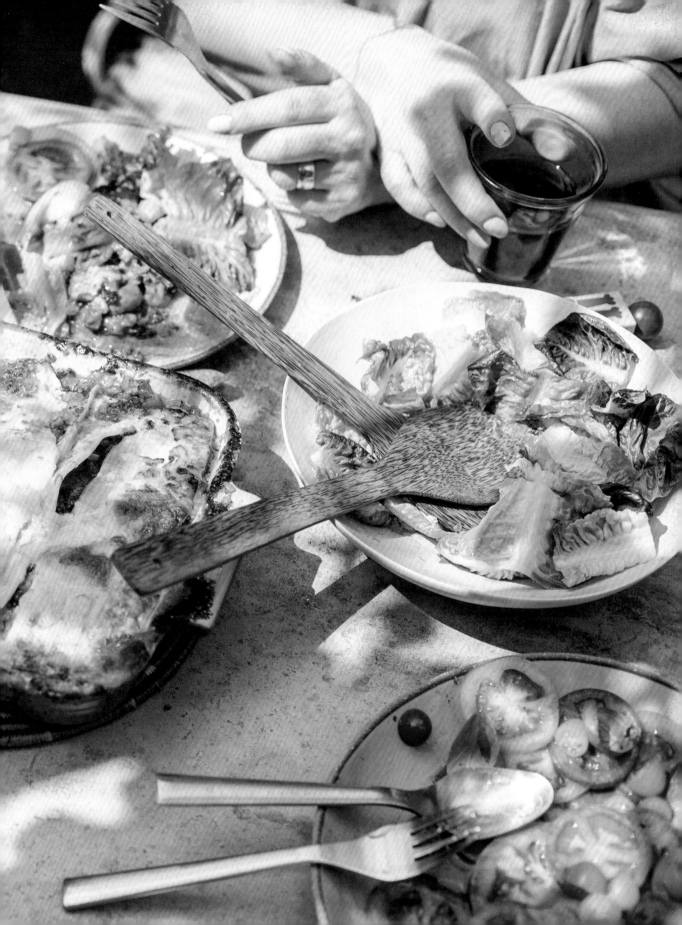

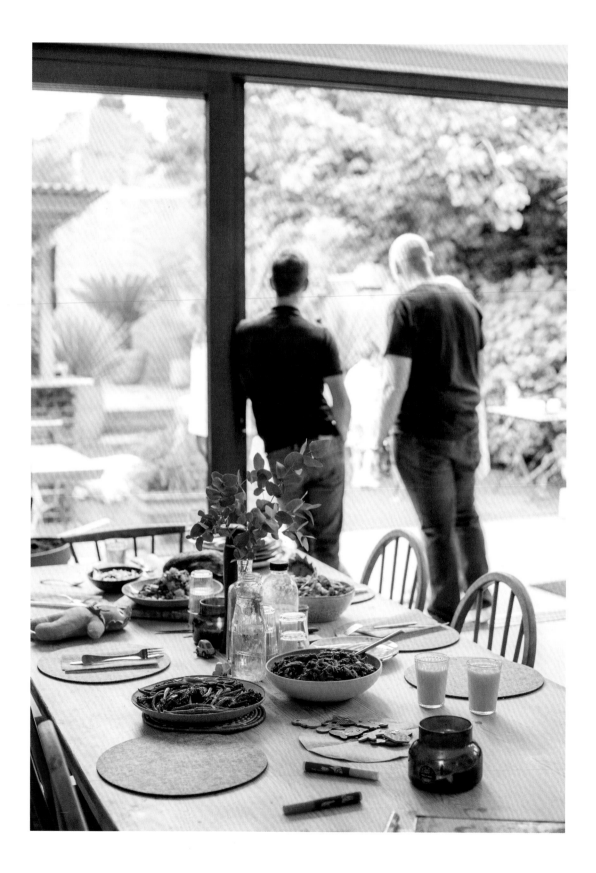

Acknowledgements

Firstly I'd like to say a massive, massive thank you to everybody at Bloomsbury and Absolute Press for sticking with me and being a part of the whole Dopamine Diet book. Jon Croft, you're a superstar as always! Big love and respect to Richard Atkinson, who believed in the vision and direction this book should go in, and who was a real help in the creative process. Hugs to Natalie Bellos, and welcome back after having your little man! Xa Shaw Stewart, you were fantastic on this, thanks so much for being such a smiley, friendly face, turning up to the shoots and going with the 'flow'! A big thank you to all the guys behind the scenes – Lena Hall, Ellen Williams, Sarah Williams and Marina Asenjo.

A massive thank you to David Eldridge and Two Associates for creating a stunning and fun book, with a 'look' that rolls through very nicely. Thank you so much Janet Illsley, the project editor. Huge respect to Lydia McPherson for the art direction, and for jumping in last minute but completely understanding what we were trying to do – girl, you're the best! And then, following on, Sarah Birks and Lauren Miller – you guys are great.

Big hugs and love to Debora Robertson for all the lengthy conversations about words and stuff. Mate, you make my life well easy! Glad the recipes worked for you. To Jennifer Hopley, who has put up with me at The Hand and Flowers for many years and is now involved in the book, advising on nutrition; well done girl, that degree was worth it! Massive thanks to Dr Rachel Gow for having a good look through the book and supporting it from a 'science' point of view!

Ta to John and Lisa at E4 Kitchen Location for lending us your house – sorry if we made a mess! Love the pizza oven.

None of this could have happened without my amazing food team: the brilliant Chris Mackett who was helped out by Jessica Mills, Holly Cochrane, Rosie Mackeane, Becs Wilkinson, Emma Laws, Pippa Leon and, of course, the forever talented bundle of energy who always makes me smile, Nicole Herft. Nicole, thank you for letting go. You've really helped make this book feel alive.

To my main man, Cristian Barnett, and his trusty sidekick Brid – you guys take the most beautiful photos. Loving the free-flow style... maybe we should do every book like this Cristian?!

To my amazing Marlow team, there are so many of you, and you are all so important! Without your determination, hard work and graft none of this would be possible. Together we grow stronger and dreams are coming true, and we will just keep pushing. There are too many people to mention, but to name but a few: Lourdes and Alan Dooley, you couple of superstars. Aaron Mulliss, Jamie May and Ollie Brown, keep smashing that kitchen in and driving it forward. Charles Beaini, Katie Gavin and Anthony Peart, thanks so much for growing with us. Nick Beardshaw, Tom De Keyser, Jonny Poynter, Claire Kreigenfeld and James Shaw, keep pushing guys, you are on a roll. And to the amazing ('you cannot start a sentence with and!') Alex Longstaff, thanks for controlling all of our lives and making the chaos that surrounds me feel like it's all in control.

Last words are to Borra Garson and Louise Leftwich at DML, and Zoe Wilmer and Amy Williams at Samphire – thanks girls!

Big love,

Tom xx

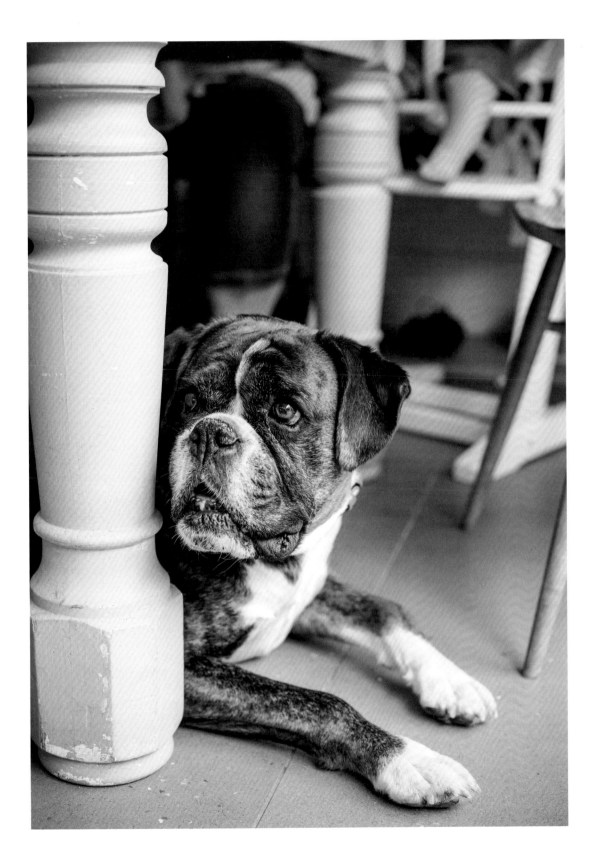

Absolute Press
An imprint of Bloomsbury Publishing Plc

50 Bedford Square
London
WC1B 3DP
UK

1385 Broadway
New York
NY 10018
USA

www.bloomsbury.com

British Library Cataloguing-in-Publication Data
A catalogue record for this book is available from the
British Library.

Library of Congress Cataloguing-in-Publication data
has been applied for.

ISBN: HB: 978-1-4729-3541-0

           ePub: 978-1-4729-3543-4

4 6 8 10 9 7 5

Project Editor: Janet Illsley
Nutritional Analysis: Jennifer Hopley BSc Hons, MSc
Design: Two Associates
Photographer: Cristian Barnett, crisbarnett.com
Food Styling: Tom Kerridge, Nicole Herft and
    Chris Mackett
Art Direction and Styling: Lydia McPherson and
    Sarah Birks
Illustrations: Two Associates
Index: Hilary Bird

Printed and bound in Italy by Graphicom

To find out more about our authors and books visit
www.bloomsbury.com. Here you will find extracts,
author interviews, details of forthcoming events and the
option to sign up for our newsletters.

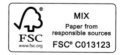

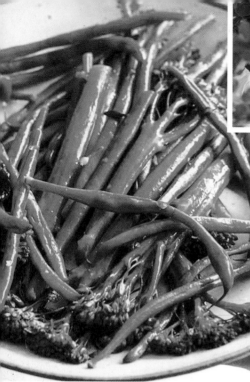
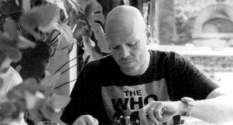
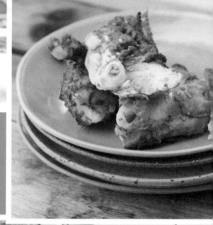
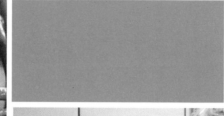
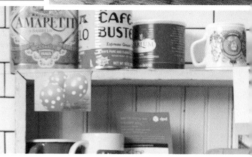
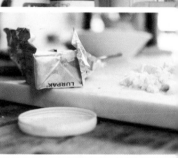

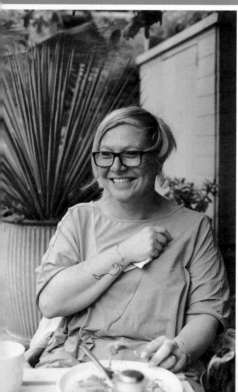
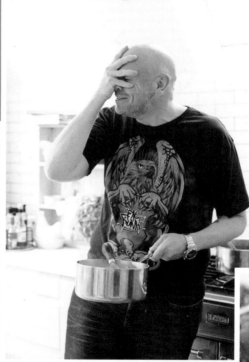
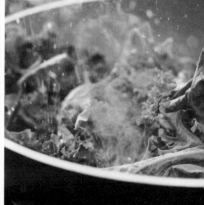